ATLAS OF
VALVULAR
CLINICAL AND PATHOLOGIC ASPECTS # HEART
DISEASE

ATLAS OF
VALVULAR
CLINICAL AND PATHOLOGIC ASPECTS
HEART
DISEASE

Guest Editors

JAMES T. WILLERSON, M.D.

Edward Randall III Professor and Chairman, Department of Internal Medicine,
University of Texas Medical School at Houston; Chief, Medical Services, Hermann Hospital;
Medical Director, Director of Cardiology Research, and Chief of Cardiology,
Texas Heart Institute, St. Luke's Episcopal Hospital, Houston, Texas

JAY N. COHN, M.D.

Professor and Head, Cardiovascular Division, Department of Medicine,
University of Minnesota Medical School, Minneapolis, Minnesota

HUGH A. MCALLISTER, JR., M.D.

Clinical Professor, Department of Pathology, Baylor College of Medicine and University
of Texas Medical School; Chief, Department of Pathology, St. Luke's Episcopal Hospital;
Chairman, Department of Cardiovascular Pathology, Texas Heart Institute,
St. Luke's Episcopal Hospital, Houston, Texas

Editors

HISAO MANABE, M.D., D.M.SC.*

President Emeritus, National Cardiovascular Center; Professor Emeritus,
Osaka University, Japan

CHIKAO YUTANI, M.D., PH.D.

Chief, Pathological Division, National Cardiovascular Center, Japan

With contributions by

**Chikao Yutani, Tsuyoshi Fujita, Makoto Takamiya, Kunio Miyatake,
Seiki Nagata, Kohei Kawazoe, Masami Imakita**

*Deceased

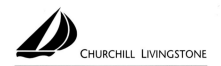
CHURCHILL LIVINGSTONE

New York, Edinburgh, London, Madrid, Melbourne, San Francisco, Tokyo

Library of Congress Cataloging-in-Publication Data

Karā atorasu benmakushō. English.
 Atlas of valvular heart disease : clinical and pathologic aspects
/ guest editors, James T. Willerson, Jay N. Cohn, Hugh A.
McAllister, Jr. ; editors, Hisao Manabe, Chikao Yutani ; with
contributions by Chikao Yutani ... [et al.].
   p.   cm.
 Tranlation of: Karā atorasu benmakushō / henshū Yutani Chikao ...
[et al.]. 1988.
   Includes bibliographical references.
   ISBN 0-443-07953-6 (alk. paper)
   1. Heart valves—Diseases—Atlases. I. Willerson, James., T.,
DATE. II. Cohn, Jay N. III. Manabe, Hisao, DATE.
IV. Yutani, Chikao. V. Title.
   [DNLM: 1. Heart Valve Diseases— pathology—atlases.   2. Diagnostic
Imaging— methods—atlases. 3. Endocarditis—pathology— atlases.
4. Heart Valve Prosthesis—atlases. WG 17 K18a 1998]
RC685.V2K3713 1998
616.1′ 25—dc21
DNLM/DLC   97-26912
for Library of Congress   CIP

Original Japanese edition published by Life Science Publishing Co., Ltd., Tokyo.
English translation rights arranged through Churchill Livingstone Japan, Tokyo.

Distributed in the United Kingdom by Churchill Livingstone, Robert Stevenson
House, 1–3 Baxter's Place, Leith Walk, Edinburgh EH1 3AF, and by associated
companies, branches, and representatives throughout the world.

Medical knowledge is constantly changing. As new information becomes available,
changes in treatment, procedures, equipment and the use of drugs become necessary.
The editors/authors/contributors and the publishers have, as far as it is possible, taken
care to ensure that the information given in this text is accurate and up to date.
However, readers are strongly advised to confirm that the information, especially with
regard to drug usage, complies with the latest legislation and standards of practice.

The Publishers have made every effort to trace the copyright holders for borrowed
material. If they have inadvertently overlooked any, they will be pleased to make the
necessary arrangements at the first opportunity.

Acquisitions Editor: *Allan Ross*
Production Editor: *Bridgett L. Dickinson*
Production Supervisor: *Laura Mosberg Cohen*
Desktop Coordinator: *Robb Quattro*
Cover Design: *Jeannette Jacobs*

Printed in Singapore

First published in 1998   7 6 5 4 3 2 1

Contributors

Chikao Yutani, M.D., Ph.D.
Director, Department of Pathology, National Cardiovascular Center, Osaka, Japan

Tsuyoshi Fujita, M.D., Ph.D.
President, Izumisano Municipal Hospital, Osaka, Japan

Makoto Takamiya, M.D., Ph.D.
Director, Department of Radiology and Nuclear Medicine, National Cardiovascular Center, Osaka, Japan

Kunio Miyatake, M.D., Ph.D., F.A.C.C.
Director, Cardiology Division of Medicine, National Cardiovascular Center, Osaka, Japan

Seiki Nagata, M.D., Ph.D.
Director, Department of Internal Medicine, Kansai Rousai Hospital, Hyogo, Japan

Kohei Kawazoe, M.D., Ph.D.
Professor, Third Department of Surgery, Iwate Medical University School of Medicine, Iwate, Japan

Masami Imakita, M.D., Ph.D.
Department of Pathology, National Cardiovascular Center, Osaka, Japan

Preface for the English Edition

This *Atlas of Valvular Heart Disease* provides a comprehensive review of valvular heart disease and its clinical and pathophysiologic aspects. The structure and function of the cardiac valves are presented. Subsequently, the various types of mitral, aortic, tricuspid, pulmonary, and prosthetic valvular disease are shown pictorially and discussed in detail. Topics covered include rheumatic valvular disease, mitral valve prolapse, infectious endocarditis, congenital abnormalities of cardiac valves, aortic valve prolapse, annuloaortic ectasia, aortitis, and prosthetic valve dysfunction. Gross photographs of different abnormalities of cardiac valves and the aorta along with representative echocardiograms help the interested reader understand valvular heart disease and provide a pictorial representation of the abnormalities that may occur. I recommend this *Atlas of Valvular Heart Disease* for any serious student of cardiovascular disease. I believe one will find it very illuminating and useful in caring for patients with these problems.

James T. Willerson, M.D.

Foreword for the Japanese Edition

Recent years have seen rapid advances in diagnostic technology for heart disease, especially in the area of diagnostic imaging techniques. As a result, much more information is now available on cardiac morphology and function. However, ultimately it is not enough simply to have access to more information; this information must be backed up by an integrated understanding of pathology and morphology. Although excellent texts are being published on the anatomy of the heart, both within Japan and overseas, something more is needed at the clinical level.

Several years ago we at the National Cardiovascular Center of Japan began working to fill this gap in the field of clinical cardiology. Fortunately, our Center since its inception has resisted departmental segregation and instead has used a cooperative interdepartmental approach to the diagnosis of heart disease. Consequently, various tests findings are investigated and discussed together to reach a diagnosis and to select the optimal therapeutic procedures for each individual case. Under this system, surgeons participate in discussions of diagnosis, and physicians specializing in internal medicine can be present at surgery to confirm clinical findings with their own eyes. Because of the many cases and the volume of data accumulated under this system, we had access to gross findings from more than 10,000 operations and 1,500 autopsies in preparing this book. As a result, we believed we were in a good position to fill the gap described above. Our planning sessions for this project included staff members who were involved in diagnostic imaging, surgery, and autopsy at the Cardiac Department of the National Cardiovascular Center. All these people worked together to develop the editorial concept on which this book is based. Our goal was to compare findings from diagnostic imaging side-by-side with gross findings from surgery and autopsy, in order to demonstrate direct organic relationships. Selecting appropriate cases from the mass of available data was a major job in itself. In addition to the photographs from surgery and autopsy, which were taken in-house, we also obtained the services of a professional photographer for extensive special photographs to show in particular the fine details of autopsy results.

Within the broad category of heart disease, we chose to focus on valvular disease because the heart valves are fundamental to the understanding of the anatomy, morphology, and function of the heart. We hope in the future to produce further volumes on congenital heart disease and cardiomyopathy. The present volume contains nearly 130 instances of valvular disease, ranging from the common to the highly distinctive. In particular, we have included sections on subjects such as prosthetic valve dysfunction, an area of growing importance in light of recent clinical trends. In all the categories presented here, we have attempted to provide a combination of clinical data and pathologic and morphologic findings from surgery and autopsy. By doing this we hope to provide information that will prove useful in understanding the pathophysiology represented in each case.

The Atlas of Valvular Heart Disease required four years from conception to completion. The resulting volume represents a new concept unlike any medical volumes now being published. Each page presents the reader with detailed visual information, and also with an artistically harmonious rendition of biologic structure and function. We hope that the result will be useful around the world, and look forward to the comments of cardiovascular specialists and of physicians and researchers in a variety of fields, including internal medicine, surgery, and pathology.

In conclusion, it gives me great pleasure to see this book published on the 10th anniversary of the National Cardiovascular Center of Japan. I would also like to express my sincere thanks to Dr. Chikao Yutani, M.D., Ph.D., Chief of the Pathology Division, National Cardiovascular Center, Japan, who took on the primary responsibility for the editing of this volume, and to all the other authors who contributed. My personal thanks go to Yukio Takadani of Life Science Publishing Co., Ltd., for his understanding and cooperation in bringing our concept to fruition, as well as to Nobumasa Takehara and Hiroyuki Hatanaka of the Editorial Department of Life Science Publishing, and also to the photographer Shuichi Kubo, who gave generously of his time and efforts in preparing the special photographs.

Hisao Manabe, M.D., D.M.Sc.

Preface for the Japanese Edition

In recent years, medicine has moved increasingly toward an explanation of pathophysiology based on cell technology and genetic engineering procedures. There is now a trend toward genetic diagnosis even at the clinical level. The field of pathology is no exception; today the spotlight is on cutting-edge research in molecular pathology. By comparison, this book offers a classical approach to valvular heart disease based on gross findings. We present it for world discussion at this time because we believe that insight into morphologic anomalies is vital for an understanding of the heart, and thus of the development of circulatory diseases. In addition, with today's rapid progress in modern diagnostic imaging, and with individual medical institutions competing to introduce ever more expensive medical equipment, there is more need than ever for a basic understanding of gross pathologic and morphologic findings in order to use this equipment for effective diagnosis. When we consider that most disease is focused in the organs and manifests as abnormal morphology, it becomes obvious that, whether in basic or clinical medical research, a practitioner who lacks a fundamental grasp of gross pathology and morphology may fail to reach an overall understanding of individual pathophysiology from an analysis based on positron computed tomography or molecular genetics. At a time like the present, when molecular biology techniques are developing rapidly, the necessity for accumulating pathologic and morphologic findings must not be overlooked.

In focusing on surgically resected valvular tissue and findings from pathologic autopsy, we have done our best to provide comparisons with findings from echocardiography and Doppler methods.

The staff of Life Science Publishing have worked diligently on the depiction of lesion sites for this book, frequently providing a professional photographer and patiently laboring to get the best possible photographs. We are very grateful for their cooperation.

Chikao Yutani
Masami Imakita

There has been dramatic progress in the development of ultrasound technology for cardiovascular applications in recent years, bringing sweeping changes to the methods applied to the diagnosis of heart disease. At present, the ultrasound techniques used for clinical cardiology applications include M-mode echocardiography, cross-sectional echocardiography, the color Doppler method, the pulse Doppler method, and the continuous-wave Doppler method. M-mode echocardiography and

cross-sectional echocardiography allow sensitive and detailed evaluation of valvular morphology and of the details of valve motion. These techniques are also useful for recording changes in ventricular or atrial size, which are frequently associated with valvular disease. The Doppler methods are well suited to evaluating regurgitant and stenotic blood flow and provide improved accuracy when evaluating the severity of these conditions. The ultrasound diagnostic techniques mentioned above are coming into broad clinical application because they are both useful and noninvasive. However, ultrasound wave imaging of the heart can obviously provide nothing more than images. In *Atlas of Valvular Heart Disease*, combining such diagnostic images with photographs from surgery and pathology, we were able to compare ultrasound findings with actual surgical and pathologic autopsy findings. By doing this, we hope to provide an increased understanding of diagnostic imaging and pathophysiology as it relates to valvular heart disease, and to further deepen the reader's knowledge of valvular disease.

Kunio Miyatake
Seiki Nagata

Conventionally, cineangiography has been considered indispensable in the diagnosis of valvular disease, and especially in the evaluation of valvular regurgitation. This role has become somewhat eclipsed by the recent development of ultrasound diagnostic methods, in particular Doppler ultrasound diagnostic methods. However, cineangiography provides a higher level of resolution, both spatial and temporal, than can be obtained with other diagnostic imaging methods. Also, because the movement of the contrast agent can be observed directly, the images are easy to interpret. Cineangiography thus remains the "gold standard" in procedures for the detailed diagnosis of lesions in valvular heart disease.

In recent years angiography has become less invasive with the development of hypo-osmotic contrast agents, "high flow" catheters, and digital imaging techniques, all of considerable diagnostic significance. The further development of cross-sectional ultrasound methods and high-speed cross-sectional imaging techniques such as cine-magnetic resonance imaging and cine-computed tomography can also be expected to provide further precision in the diagnosis of valvular heart disease.

We have always taken pains to keep up with modern surgical techniques. However, while reviewing and reconsidering pathologic and surgical specimens and surgical color photographs in the process of assembling this book, we were able to fill in details that had gone unnoticed in the operating room. We feel sure that this volume will be useful in deepening the reader's understanding of valvular heart disease, and will provide a major contribution to the ability to interpret medical images of valvular disease.

Makoto Takamiya

The intraoperative photographs assembled for this book were taken successively whenever an opportunity presented itself during one of our surgeries. From this "hand-made" record we have selected the clearest photographs for presentation here. The comments on surgical intervention in the text are based on our own surgical experience and focus primarily on surgical technique.

During surgical preparation in cases of valvular heart disease, the surgeon first studies a variety of diagnostic images in order to develop a clear picture of the movement of the valve in the beating heart. The surgeon then considers what type of surgery would be appropriate in this case, and the best sequence of procedures to use. We have tried to reproduce in this *Atlas of Valvular Heart Disease* photographs and images that will communicate to the reader the day-to-day process within the minds of surgeons as they go about this work.

Tsuyoshi Fujita
Kohei Kawazoe

Contents

I
Structure and Function of Cardiac Valves

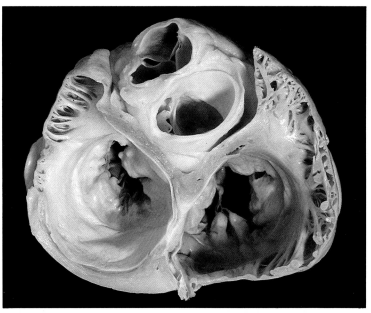

Heart of a 51-year-old man with no known history of heart disease. In this cross-sectional view, all four valves are visible.

The human heart weighs approximately 300 to 350 g at autopsy, with weights 20 to 30 g greater in men than in women. The heart is generally considered to be about the same size as the person's fist.

Within the mediastinum, the cardiac apex is directed to the left and is positioned on the posterior wall of the diaphragm. However, generally in pathologic examination of the heart, the cardiac apex is positioned vertically (Fig. 1) in order to observe structures such as the atria, ventricles, and various major blood vessels and to evaluate the condition of the heart valves. When the heart is viewed in this way from above (Fig. 2), the pulmonary artery is anterior and the aorta is posterior, with the atria and atrial auricles visible to the left and right.

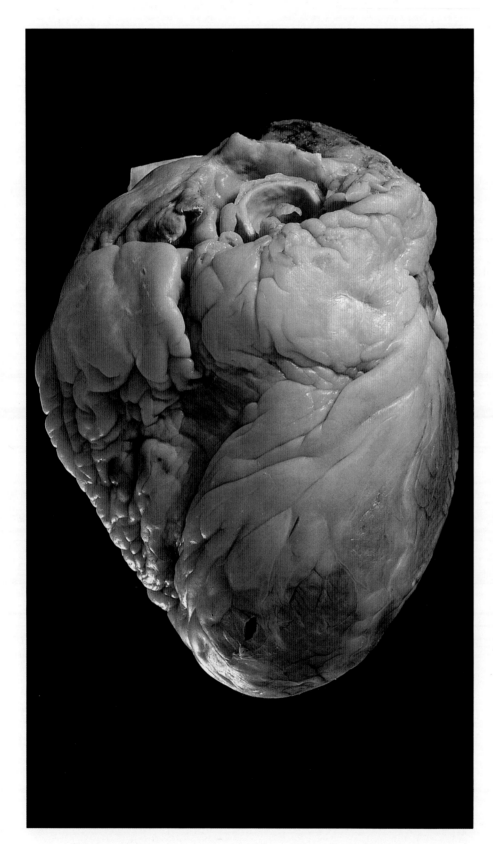

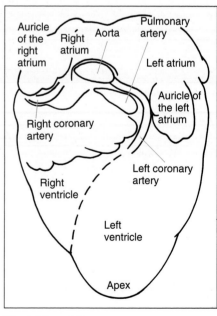

FIG. 1 Normal front view.

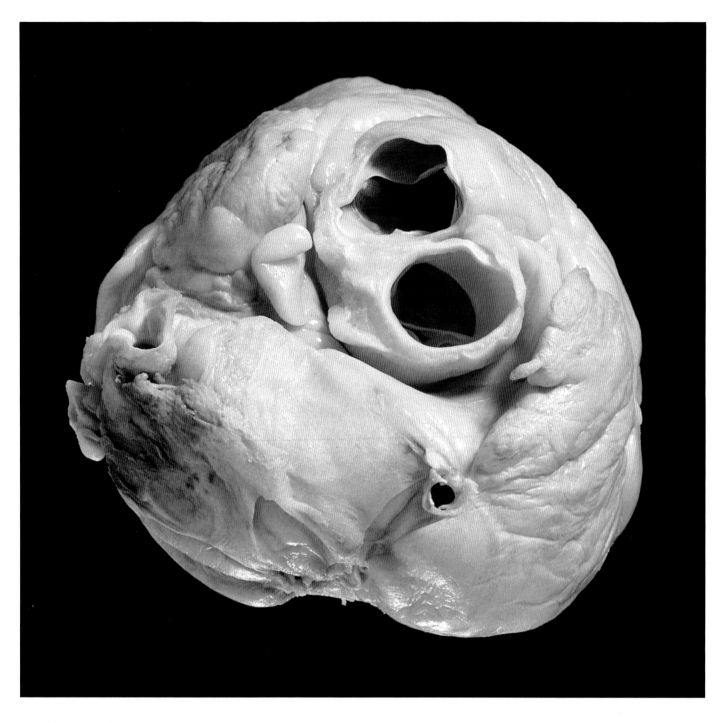

FIG. 2 View from above.

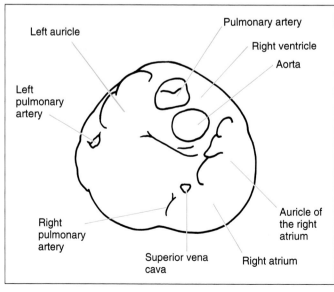

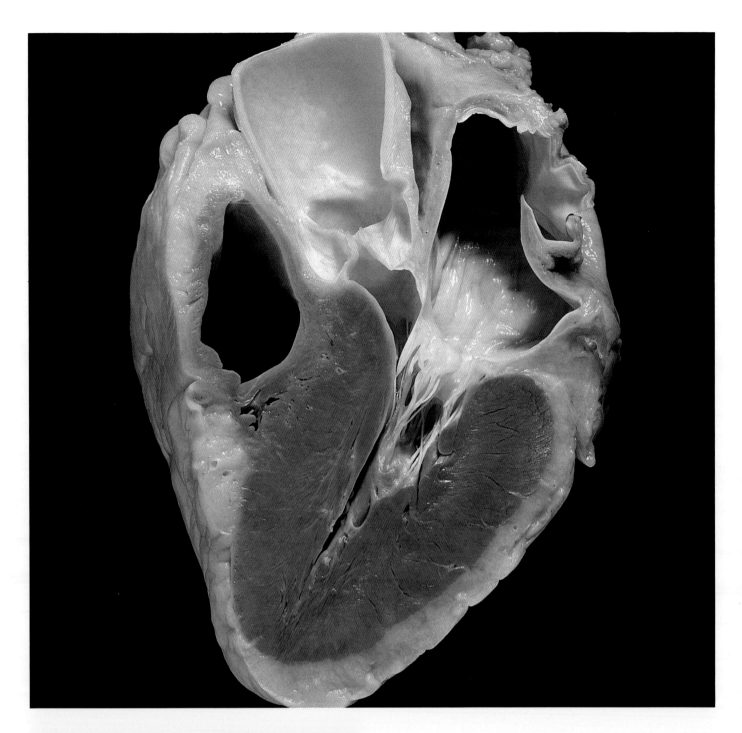

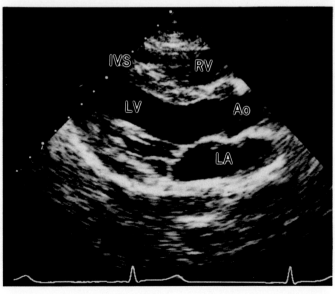

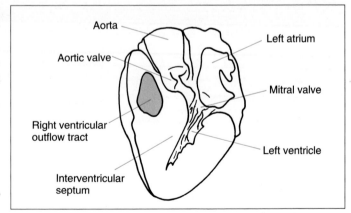

FIG. 3 Heart of a 74-year-old woman with no known history of heart disease (cross-section, including the mitral valve and the aortic valve), with the corresponding cross-sectional echocardiogram. (Ao, aorta; IVS, interventricular septum; LA, left atrium; LV, left ventricle; RV, right ventricle.)

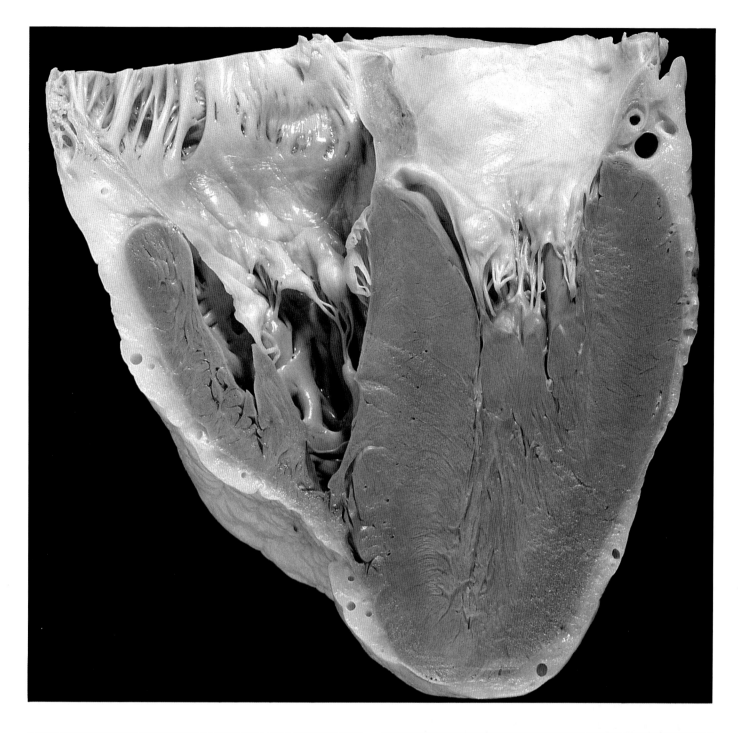

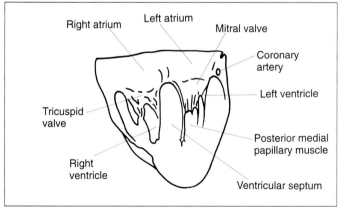

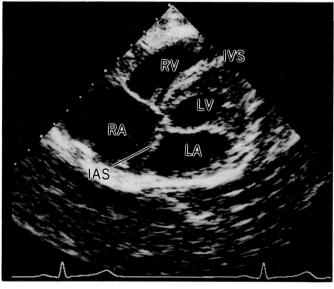

FIG. 4 Heart of a 51-year-old man with no known history of heart disease (cross-section through the center of the tricuspid and mitral valves), with the corresponding cross-sectional echocardiogram. (IAS, interatrial septum; IVS, interventricular septum; LA, left atrium; LV, left ventricle; RA, right atrium; RV, right ventricle.)

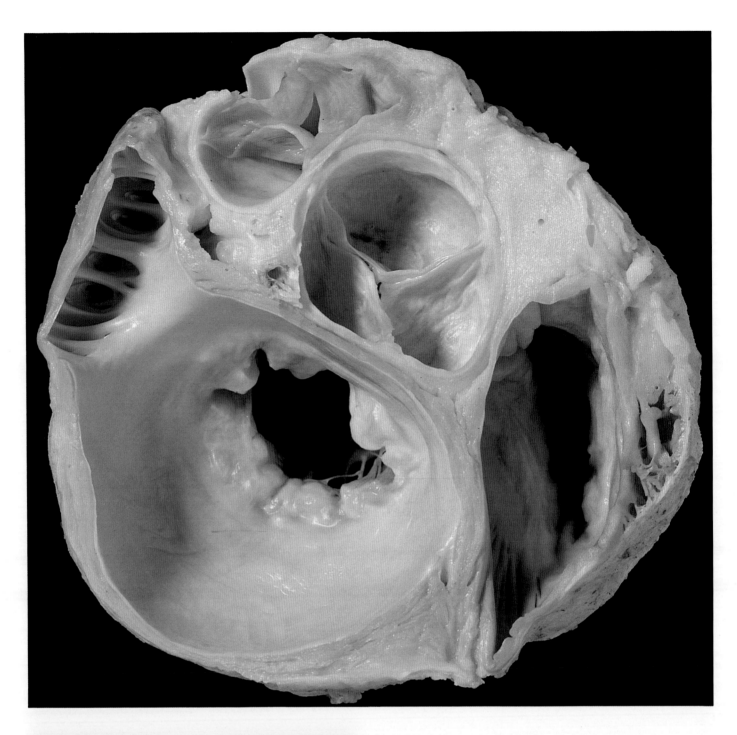

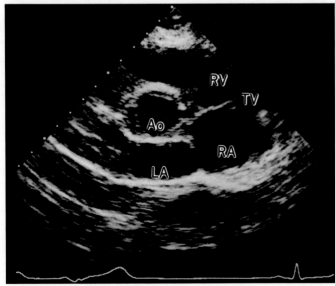

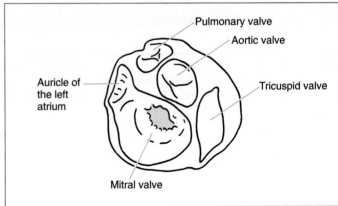

FIG. 5 Heart of a 68-year-old woman with a history of angina pectoris (horizontal cross-section at the level of the aortic valve ring), with the corresponding cross-sectional echocardiogram. (Ao, aorta; LA, left atrium; RA, right atrium; RV, right ventricle; TV, tricuspid valve.)

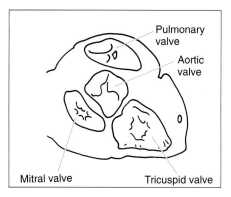

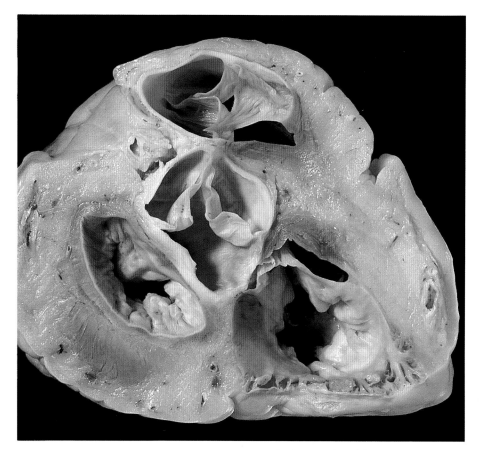

FIG. 6 Horizontal cross-section at the level of the mitral valve ring (systole).

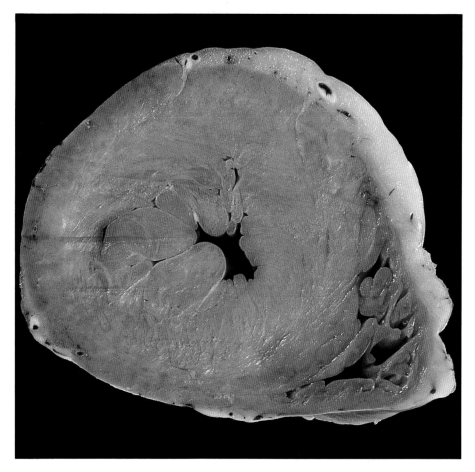

FIG. 7 Horizontal cross-section of the papillary muscle, mid-level (systole).

Mitral Valve

Of the four valves in the heart, only the mitral valve is bicuspid; the remaining three are configured as tricuspid valves. Understanding the structure and function of the mitral valve requires that we consider not only the valve itself, but also the tissues around it that provide support. These supportive tissue structures are made up of the valve leaflets, the chordae tendineae, the papillary muscle, and the valve ring (annulus) and are designated generally as mitral valve supporting tissue.

When pressure within the left atrium exceeds the pressure in the left ventricle, the mitral valve leaflets open in the direction of the ventricle. When the pressure within the ventricle beneath these valve leaflets is elevated during systole, the leaflets close, preventing regurgitation from the ventricle into the atrium. This rapid series of movements is coordinated with contraction and expansion of the left ventricular myocardium. Contractions of the papillary muscles, which are part of the ventricular myocardium, are communicated through tension on the chordae tendineae, causing the valve to open and close smoothly.

Figure 8 shows the mitral valve as viewed from the left atrium during left ventricular systole, when the valve is closed. The anterior leaflet appears to be largely formed through the base of the atrium. Detailed examination of the crescent-shaped posterior leaflet shows it to consist of three smaller leaflets. The anterior and posterior leaflets occlude for a width of approximately 5 mm from the free margin (Figs. 8 to 10). As pressure in the left ventricle rises, the valve closes more firmly.

When we view the open mitral valve after dissection of the valve ring (Figs. 11 to 13), the anterior leaflet takes on a semicircular form and the posterior leaflet is elongated. From the fixed region of the valve to the free margin, the length of the anterior leaflet is approximately three times greater than that of the posterior leaflet, although the valve area is nearly identical (Fig. 11). The fixed region of the posterior leaflet consists of the fibrous valve ring. One portion of the anterior leaflet is continuous with the aortic valve, while another portion connects to the membrane of the interventricular septum. These portions play an important role in the function of the anterior leaflet, serving to separate inflow and outflow of blood through the left ventricle (Fig. 12).

These two leaflets, anterior and posterior, close medially and laterally at the commissure, where fan-shaped chordae tendineae can be identified by the naked eye. Fusion does not normally occur in this area. The chordae tendineae insert into two papillary muscles. An average of 24 chordae tendineae are connected to the papillary muscles and branch into 120 small chordae tendineae, which attach to the valve leaflets to form the rough zone. Where these chordae tendineae branch from the papillary muscle, they are termed the *primary*, *secondary*, and *tertiary* chordae tendineae (Fig. 13). Inflow from the left atrium passes through a chamber bounded by these chordae tendineae. Understandably, thickening of the chordae tendineae, as occurs in rheumatic mitral valve disease, interferes with this smooth blood flow.

The two papillary muscles are divided respectively into the posterior medial and anterior lateral groups. There is considerable variation in the number of small papillary muscles, and their position may vary from one case to the next (Figs. 9 to 11). Normally the posterior medial papillary muscle is supplied with blood by the right coronary artery, while the anterior lateral papillary muscle is supplied by the left circumflex artery.

As viewed by the naked eye, the mitral valve leaflets can be considered in three sections. The area where the chordae tendineae attaches is termed the *rough zone*, the region near attachment to the fibrous valve ring is termed the *basal zone*, and the intermediate region, transparent in normal valves, is termed the *clear zone*.

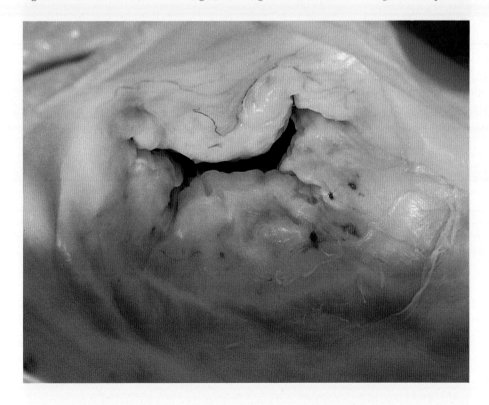

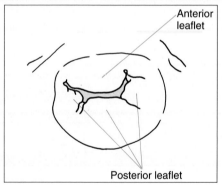

FIG. 8 Mitral valve of a 72-year-old woman viewed from the atrial side. The patient was hypertensive; death resulted from cerebral infarction.

Valve structure at the cellular level clearly shows a fibrous layer (the pars fibrosa) directly beneath the endothelial cells on the surface of the atrium. Collagen fibers and elastic fibers are also abundantly present. The rough myxomatous structure present in the central region (the pars spongiosa) is sponge-like in appearance. There is another fibrous layer on the ventricular surface, and multiple layers of elastic fiber are visible extending to the endothelial cells.

In subjects 20 years of age or younger, the mitral valve is generally quite transparent, darkening to opacity in patients 50 years of age or older. This area is normally exposed to high pressure, and fatty deposits are frequently visible on the ventricular side of the anterior leaflet, but these findings are rarely pathologic (Fig. 9).

After 70 years of age, nodular thickening at the closing margin is seen on the atrial surface of the mitral valve; this thickening is attributed to physiologic trauma (Fig. 11). In particular, hooding is frequently seen on the atrial side of the posterior leaflet, between the chordae tendineae on the free margin.

Aging brings an increase in the frequency of calcification of the mitral valve ring. This point is discussed further in subsequent pages.

FIG. 9 Normal funnel-shaped structure of the mitral valve of a 49-year-old man. The patient had a history of hypertension and gout and died of cerebral hemorrhage.

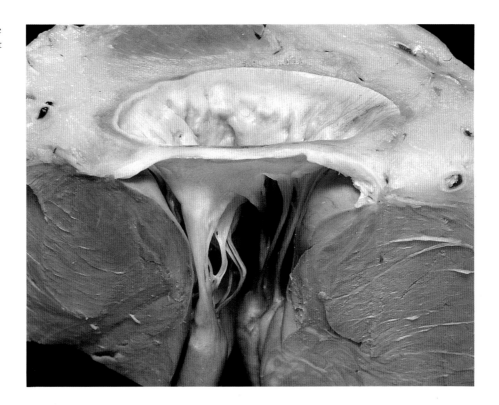

FIG. 10 Resected mitral valve from the same patient shown in Fig. 8. The anterior leaflet of the mitral valve is visible on the posterior surface. On the left is the anterior lateral papillary muscle group; on the right is the posterior medial papillary muscle group.

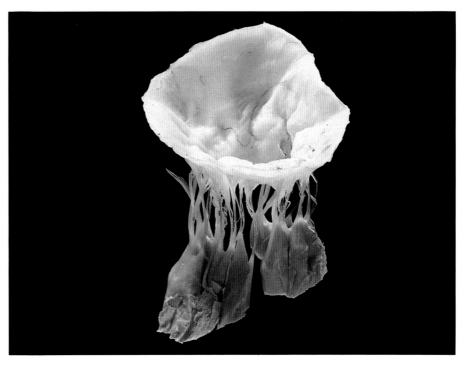

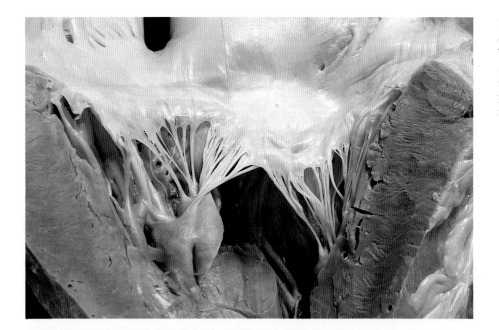

FIG. 11 View of the mitral valve of a 70-year-old man dissected through the posterior wall. The man died of a ruptured abdominal aortic aneurysm. The anterior leaflet is visible on the right and the posterior leaflet on the left. The papillary muscle group on the left is the anterior lateral papillary muscle group.

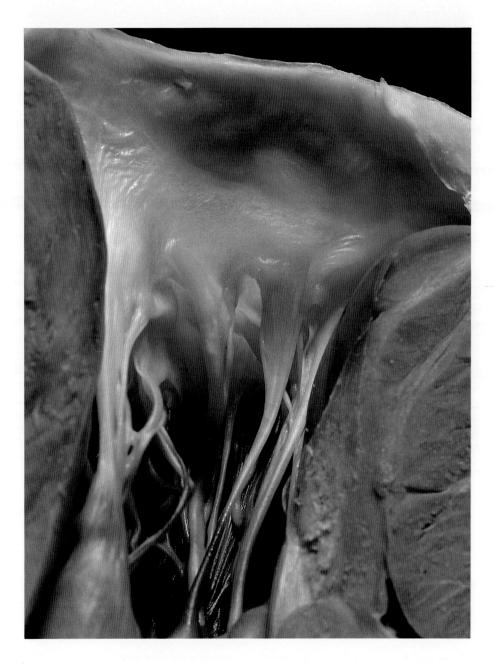

FIG. 12 View from the ventricular side of the anterior leaflet of the mitral valve of a 49-year-old man. The patient had a history of hypertension; death resulted from cerebral hemorrhage.

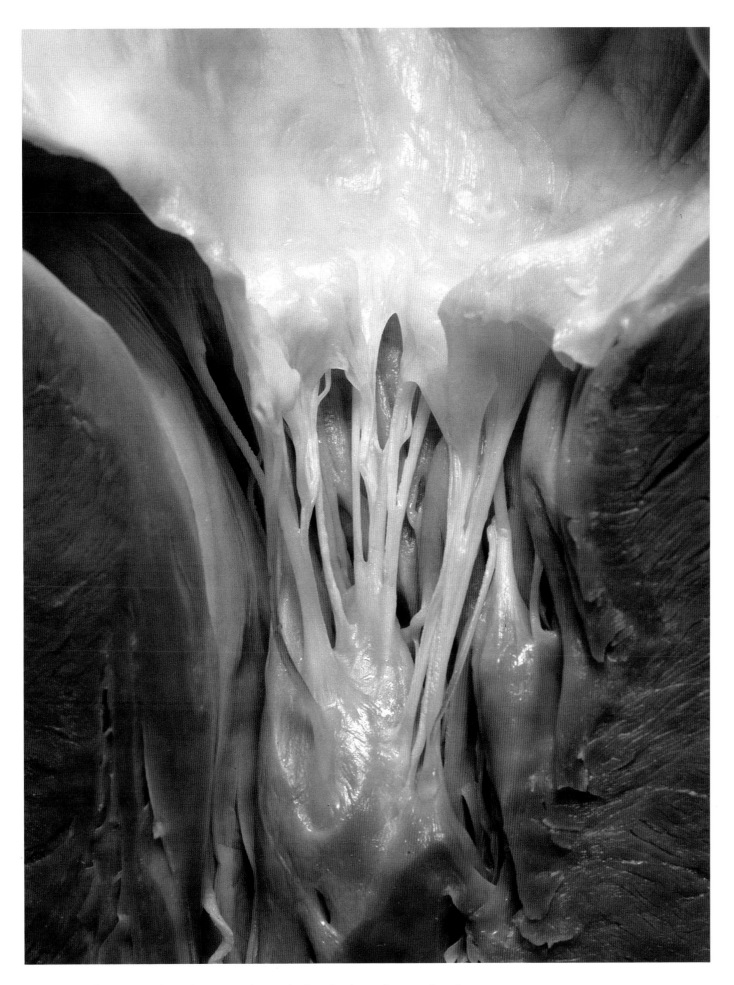

FIG. 13 View showing the relationships among the mitral valve, chordae tendineae, and papillary muscles of a 74-year-old woman who died of a ruptured cerebral aneurysm. The anterior leaflet is visible on the left and the posterior leaflet on the right. The papillary muscle in the center is the anterior lateral papillary muscle group.

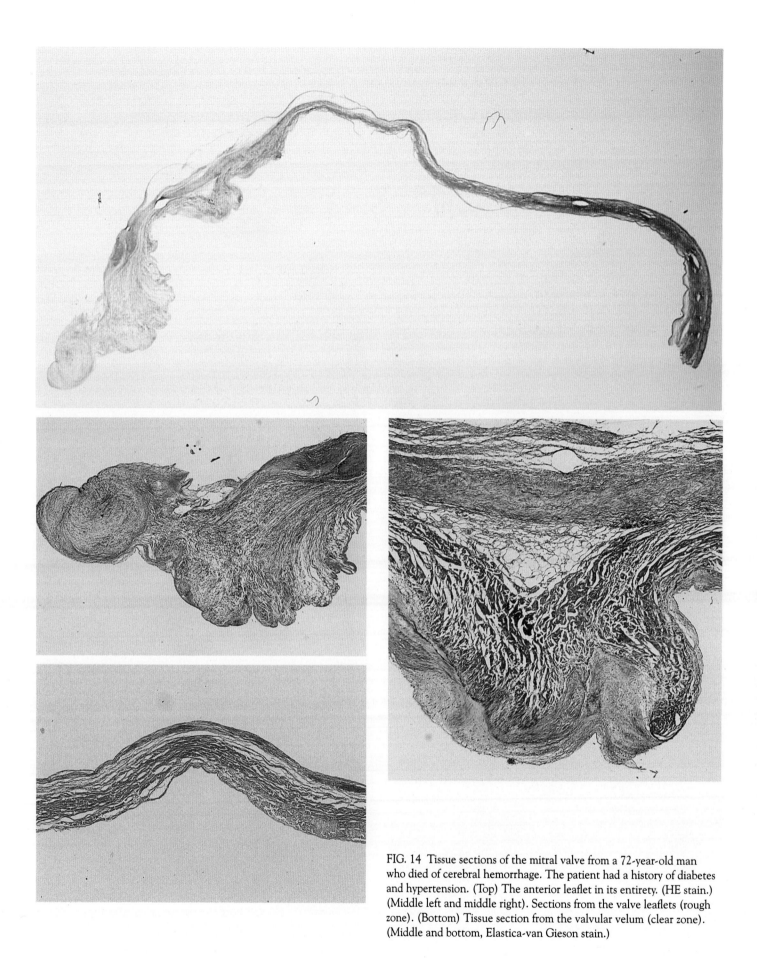

FIG. 14 Tissue sections of the mitral valve from a 72-year-old man who died of cerebral hemorrhage. The patient had a history of diabetes and hypertension. (Top) The anterior leaflet in its entirety. (HE stain.) (Middle left and middle right). Sections from the valve leaflets (rough zone). (Bottom) Tissue section from the valvular velum (clear zone). (Middle and bottom, Elastica-van Gieson stain.)

Aortic Valve

The aortic valve, like the pulmonary valve, contains three semilunar cusps. These cusps form the sinuses of Valsalva, with the aortic wall as the outer side. The three valve leaflets are termed the *left coronary cusp, right coronary cusp,* and *noncoronary cusp,* depending on their position with regard to the openings of the coronary arteries. During systole, these sinuses of Valsalva contract and send blood into the coronary arteries. At the upper margin of the sinuses of Valsalva, at the transition to the origin of the aorta, a knob-like protuberance can be observed. Approximately two-thirds of the aortic valve ring is connected to the muscular portion of the ventricular septum, while the remaining one-third is connected to the anterior leaflet of the mitral valve.

When pressure rises within the left ventricle, the three valve leaflets move toward the aortic walls of their respective sinuses, equalizing the pressure differential between the interior of the left ventricle and the aortic lumen. If the pressure at the base of the aorta exceeds left intraventricular pressure, the valve leaflets close the lumen to prevent regurgitation. There are two important elements that support this function. The first is the semilunar shape of each valve leaflet, and the second is the way in which the free margins overlap in closing the lumen. At closure, the total area, as formed by the free margins of the aortic valve leaflets, is approximately 10% greater than the area of the base of the aorta. Central to the irregularities that are visible on the free margins are small nodules termed the *Arantius nodules.*

A comparison of valve leaflet areas shows that the right coronary cusp is normally the largest, followed by the noncoronary cusp, with the left coronary cusp accounting for the smallest area. The histologic structure of the aortic valve is very simple. The central portion of the valve is a rough myxomatous structure having a sponge-like appearance and termed the *pars spongiosa.* It is bordered on either side by the pars fibrosa, consisting of dense collagen fibers. Surfaces that come into contact with the blood are coated with endothelial cells. Similarly to the mitral valve, the aortic valve leaflets do not contain nutrient blood vessels.

FIG. 15 Aortic valve viewed from the aorta of a 72-year-old man. The left coronary cusp is visible to the upper left, the right coronary cusp to the upper right, and the noncoronary cusp below.

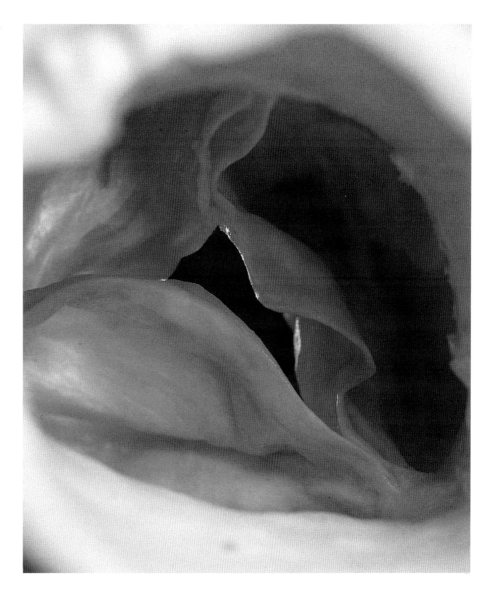

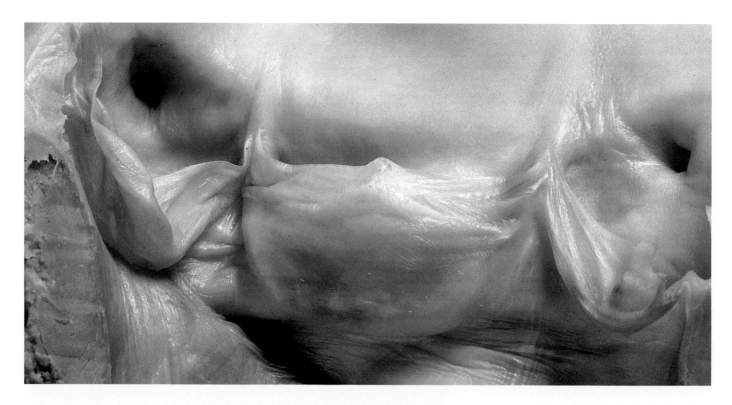

FIG. 16 View of the aortic valve of a 42-year-old man after dissection of the left ventricular outflow tract. From the left, the right coronary cusp (the opening of the right coronary artery is visible), the noncoronary cusp, and the left coronary cusp (the opening of the left coronary artery is visible) is shown.

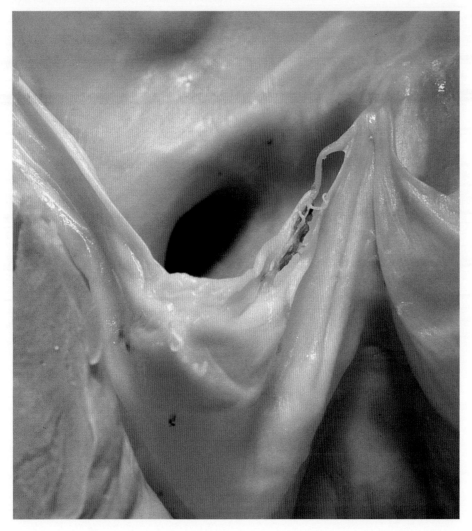

FIG. 17 Fenestrated lesion of a 70-year-old man. Fenestration is visible in the right coronary cusp.

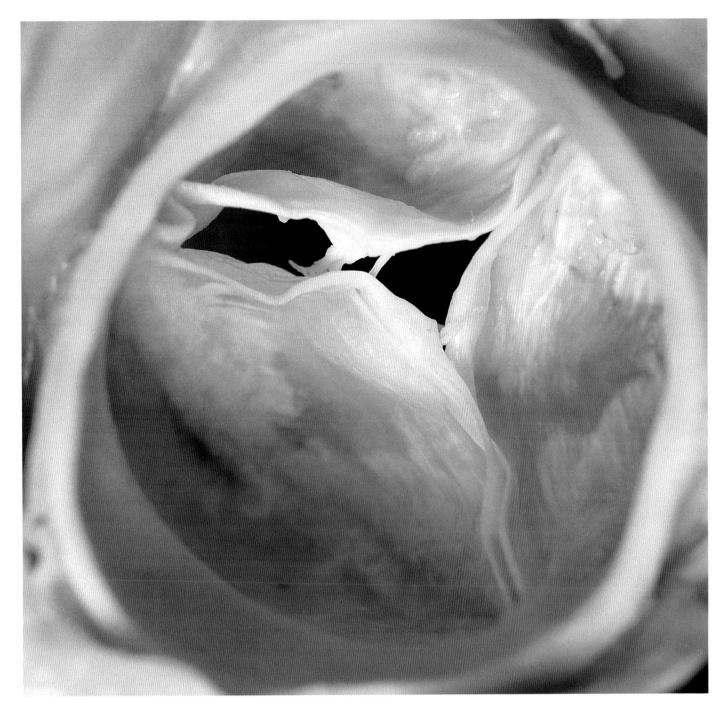

FIG. 18 Lambl's excrescences (projections) of a 73-year-old man. A view from the aortic side of the aortic valve shows changes as a result of aging. The valve leaflets show xanthomatous and calcified deposits, with Lambl's excrescences near the closing margins.

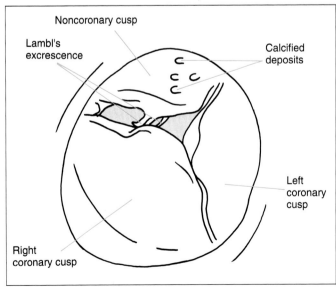

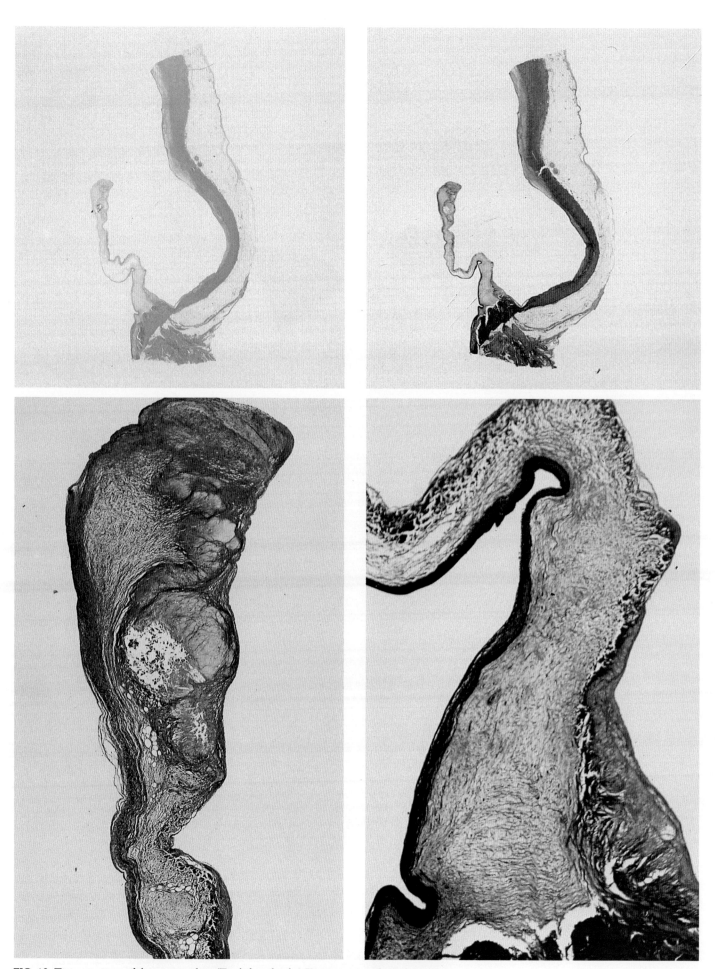

FIG. 19 Tissue sections of the aortic valve. (Top left and right) Tissue sections from the aortic valve and the sinuses of Valsalva. (Top left, HE stain; top right; Elastica-van Gieson stain.) (Bottom left and bottom right) Microscopic sections of aortic valve tissue. (Elastica-van Gieson stain.) The central portion of the valvular tissue consists of spongy tissue (pars spongiosa), while on both sides the valve is made up of fibrous layers (pars fibrosa) containing elastic fibers.

Tricuspid Valve

The basic structure and function of the tricuspid valve are the same as in the mitral valve. The orifice of the tricuspid valve is larger than in the mitral valve and is positioned nearly on the sagittal cross-section; blood from the right atrium flows downward in a left anterior direction. The valve leaflets are thinner than in the mitral valve and highly transparent; three nonhomogeneous leaflets can be identified. The anterior leaflet is the largest, reaching from the infundibulum toward the inferior lateral wall of the right ventricle. The septal leaflet extends between the membranous and muscular portions of the ventricular septum. The posterior leaflet, normally the smallest, is attached to the posterior inferior wall. Three papillary muscle groups are normally present (Fig. 21). The anterior papillary muscle is the largest, is positioned at the commissure of the anterior and posterior leaflets, and originates from the moderator band and the anterior lateral wall. The posterior papillary muscle lies below the commissure of the posterior leaflet and septal leaflet. The septal papillary muscle is small, and originates from the infundibulum. In some cases this muscle is undetectable, and the chordae tendineae insert directly into the infundibulum.

Mitral valve prolapse is accompanied in 30% of cases by a similar prolapse of the tricuspid valve.

In patients suffering from a variety of lung diseases that involve elevation of the pulmonary arterial pressure, including primary pulmonary hypertension, chronic bronchitis, and pulmonary emphysema, doming of the tricuspid valve and enlargement of the valve leaflets are frequently observed and may cause clinical regurgitation. On closer observation, ulcer formation may be noted on the anterior leaflet surface along the inflow tract. This condition is observed in approximately 6% of all autopsied hearts, but is found very frequently as a complication of pulmonary disease (97% of cases).

Newborns and infants often (approximately 56% of cases) show small cysts containing blood on the atrial surface of the tricuspid valve; these are termed *bloody cysts*.

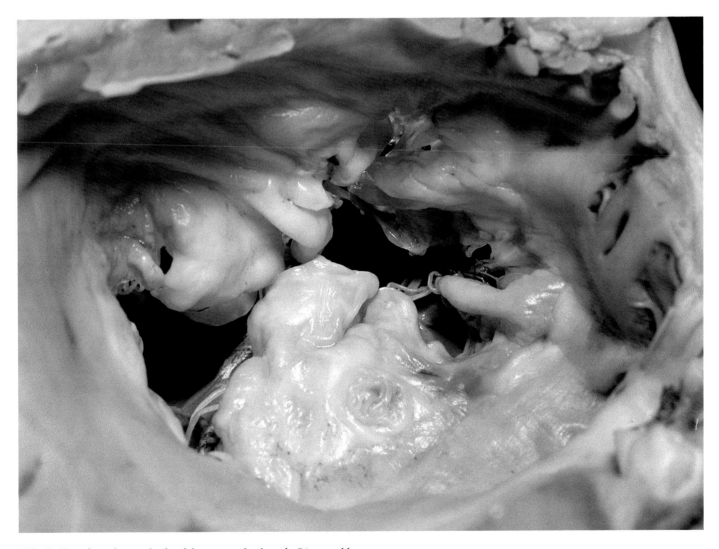

FIG. 20 View from the atrial side of the tricuspid valve of a 74-year-old woman. The septal leaflet is visible in the lower part of the figure, the anterior cusp in the upper left, and the posterior cusp in the upper right.

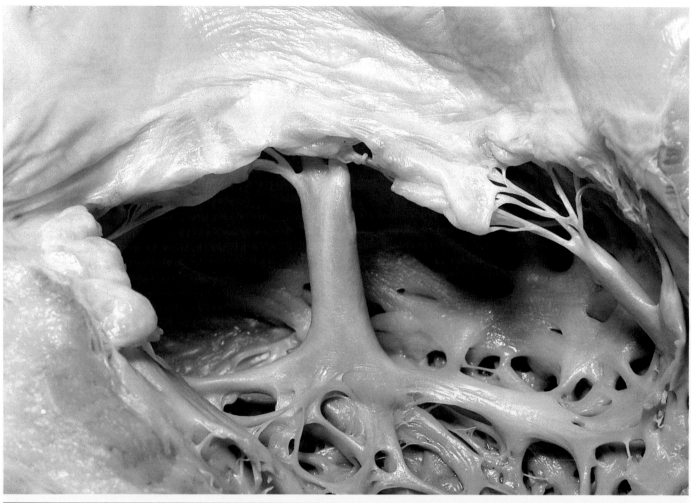

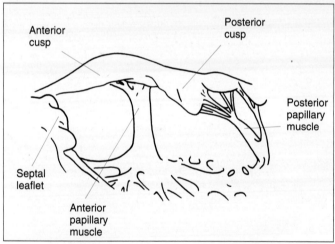

Anterior
cusp

Posterior
cusp

Posterior
papillary
muscle

Septal
leaflet

Anterior
papillary
muscle

FIG. 21 View of the tricuspid valve after dissection of the posterior wall of the right ventricle. The anterior leaflet is visible to the upper left, and the posterior leaflet to the upper right.

Pulmonary Valve

The pulmonary valve is similar in basic structure and function to the aortic valve. It is positioned forward, left, and somewhat above the aortic valve, and consists of three semilunar valve leaflets termed the *anterior cusp,* the *right cusp,* and the *leaf cusp* (Figs. 23 and 24).

In pulmonary hypertension, the valve leaflets may thicken and become fibrous. Fenestrated lesions may also occur with aging, just as in the aortic valve. Very rarely the pulmonary valve may be bicuspid or tetracuspid.

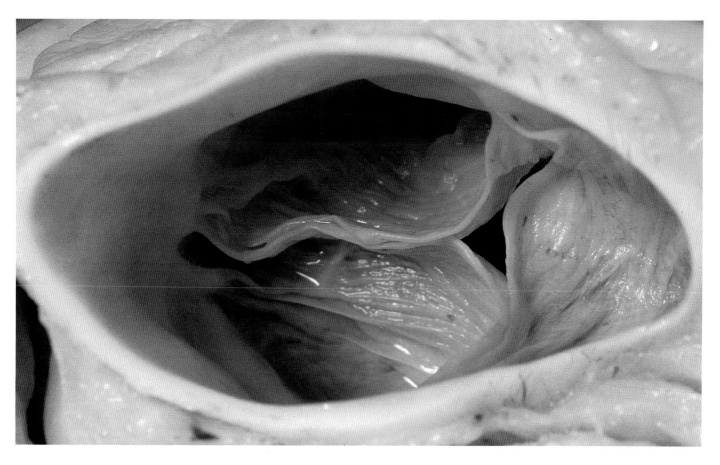

FIG. 22 View of the pulmonary valve seen from the pulmonary artery of a 42-year-old man. The upper side of the figure shows the anterior (ventral) surface.

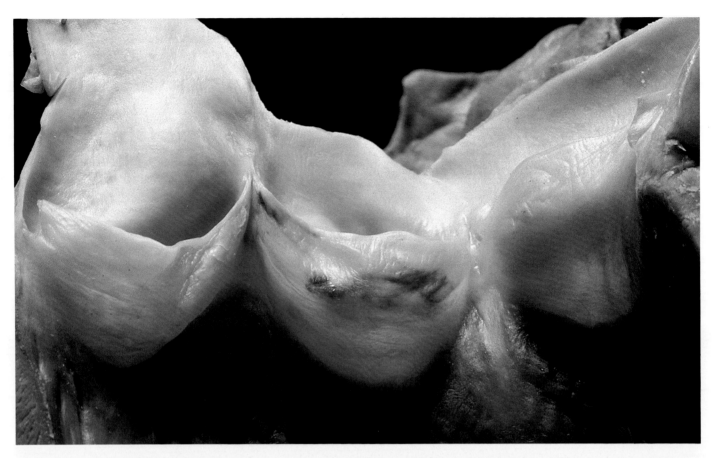

FIG. 23 View of the pulmonary valve following dissection of the right ventricular outflow tract, of the same case shown in Fig. 22. From the left, the figure shows the anterior cusp, the right cusp, and the left cusp.

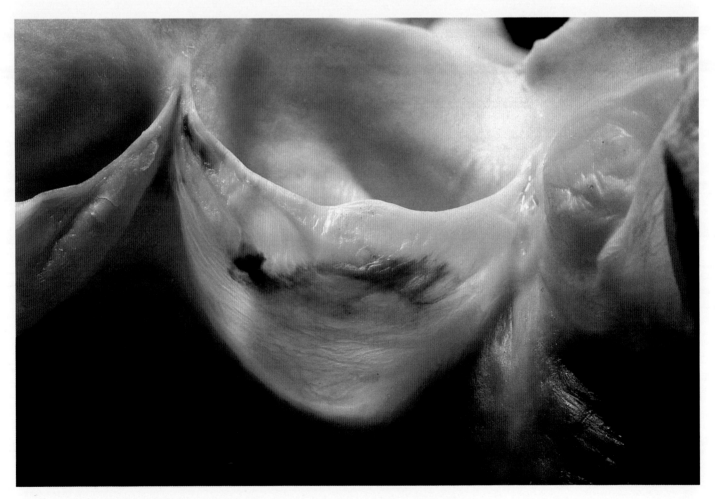

FIG. 24 Enlargement of the right cusp of the pulmonary valve of the same case shown in Fig. 22.

Valvular System and Myocardial Contraction

From the end of diastole (Fig. 25A) through the isovolumetric phase of systole (Fig. 25B), closure of the mitral and tricuspid valves proceeds continuously in the sequential closure mechanisms described in no. 1 to 3 below. At the same time, from the end of diastole, the activity described in no. 4 below occurs in parallel with no. 1 to 3.

1. When the jet of blood flowing into the ventricle as a result of atrial contraction suddenly ceases, a negative pressure occurs on the inner aspect (atrial side) of the valve leaflets, causing these leaflets to be drawn toward each other. The valve leaflets come together first in the area near the valve ring and last at the valve margins. This minimizes regurgitation due to valve closure. At the same time, blood following into the ventricle forms an eddy on the dorsal (ventricular) aspect of the valve leaflets, which acts to press the leaflets closed.

2. The papillary muscles begin to contract very early in ventricular systole, before the rest of the ventricular wall. This pulls the valve leaflets toward the cardiac apex and brings the valve margins closer together.

3. During the isovolumetric phase in early ventricular systole, as soon as intraventricular pressure exceeds atrial pressure, the atrioventricular valve is pushed up toward the atrium and the valve closes. This mechanism alone produces a certain amount of regurgitation accompanying valve closure.

4. The atrioventricular valve ring on the free wall side demonstrates repeated sphincter-like contractions. During the last stage of ventricular contraction, the annular area is constricted by approximately 30% in comparison to the maximum open orifice. However, two-thirds of this is due to atrial contraction. Most annular contraction occurs immediately before valve closure, bringing the entire body of the valve leaflets into close proximity.

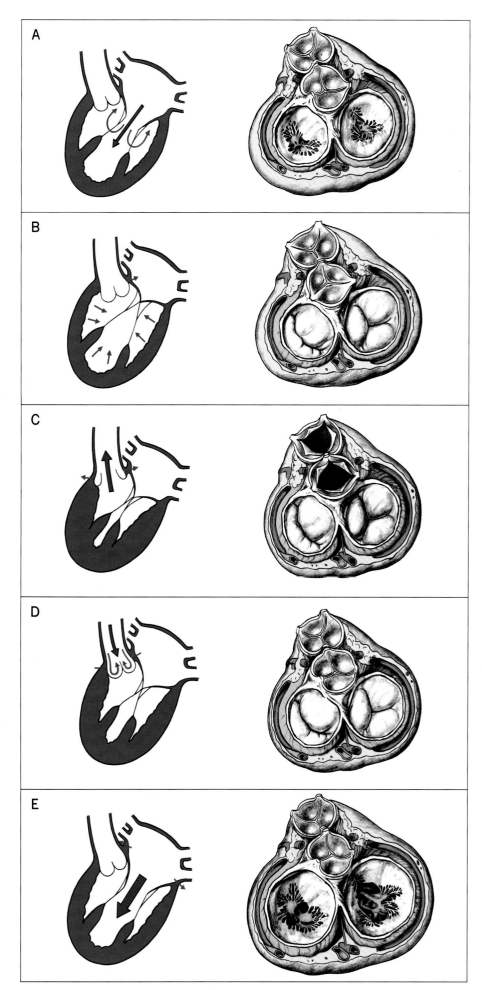

FIG. 25 Valve closure and myocardial contractions.

The aortic valve opens by progressive dilation beginning at the base of the aorta in the early stage of ventricular contraction, immediately before blood is ejected into the aorta. With progressive dilation at the base of the aorta, each commissure is pushed laterally, and the valve leaflets are pulled to the outside; the orifice of the aortic valve takes on a stellar configuration (Fig. 25B). As the heart moves into the ejection phase (Fig. 25C) and the valve ring continues to expand, the orifice assumes a triangular shape with the length of a valve leaflet making up each leg of the triangle. When the blood flows rapidly through the aortic valve, the valve leaflets are pressed farther to the outside, and the orifice assumes a circular configuration.

In isovolumetric relaxation (Fig. 25D), blood flow is suddenly interrupted. A negative pressure wave from within the aorta then pulls the valve leaflets toward the center, initiating closure of the aortic valve. Regurgitation within the sinuses of Valsalva pushes the valve leaflets from the rear toward the center, while the drop in intraventricular pressure produces constriction of the valve ring, further contributing to valve closure. The opening and closing mechanisms for the pulmonary valve are nearly identical to those for the aortic valve.

As blood flows into the ventricle, both the mitral valve and the tricuspid valve begin to open. The valve leaflets rapidly attain their maximum open position (Fig. 25E) at the beginning of diastole (period of rapid filling). After this rapid filling stage is completed, the valve leaflets return to a semiclosed position in relatively close proximity to each other. They reopen temporarily for inflow from the subsequent atrial contraction, after which they close completely. If the heart rate is high at this point, the atrial contraction is continuous with the rapid filling stage, and no semiclosure is evidenced.

II
Mitral
Valvular Disease

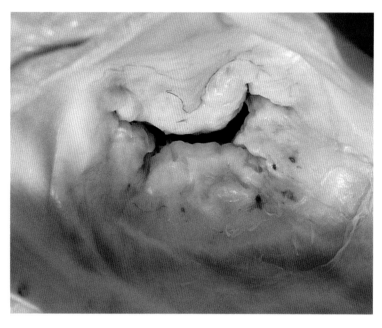

Mitral valve of a 72-year-old woman with a history of hypertension.

Rheumatic Valvular Disease

Rheumatic fever, a systemic inflammatory connective tissue reaction secondary to infection by group A hemolytic streptococcus, preferentially affects the heart valve to produce a variety of valvular diseases. Of the four cardiac valves, rheumatic fever involves the mitral valve alone in 62%, the aortic valve alone in 5%, and both valves in 33% of cases.

Rheumatic fever arises primarily through an autoimmune mechanism as a sequela of group A hemolytic streptococcus infection and is accompanied by some form of inflammation in approximately 60% to 70% of cases. Submiliary granulomas, termed *Aschoff bodies,* are also sometimes present.

In the early stages of this disease, the valve leaflets become edematous and monocytic infiltration is evidenced. Subsequently, the valve leaflets gradually thicken and lose their transparency, excrescences (projections) form at the closing margin of the valve, and neovascularization results in valvular thickening.

As damage progresses, increasing granulation and fibrotic changes produce valvular thickening, shortening of the chordae tendineae, and deformation of the valve ring, resulting in functional valvular stenosis and insufficiency. Changes in the endocardium within the left atrium contribute greatly to enlargement of the left atrium and formation of left intra-atrial thrombi.

It is not uncommon for patients with a past history of rheumatic fever to show the first symptoms of valvular heart disease, especially mitral stenosis, 10 years or more after infection. Conditions related to valvular insufficiency are also frequently discovered in patients having no past history of rheumatic fever. In cases of cardiac insufficiency due to rheumatic valvular disease in its clinically chronic stage, particularly where this insufficiency is caused by morphologic anomalies, patients should be considered as candidates for surgical intervention.

Mitral Stenosis

Mitral stenosis occurs as a result of a combination of changes, including thickening of the valve leaflets, fibrotic changes and calcification, and adhesions and shortening of the chordae tendineae, as well as from adhesions in the commissures. Underlying abnormalities related to valve function involve obstruction of blood flow through the mitral valve and loss of valve mobility.

The normal mitral valve orifice is approximately 6 cm^2 in area. There is little hemodynamic impairment when the valve orifice is 2 cm^2 or above, and daily activities can be carried out at 1.6 cm^2 or above. Patients become symptomatic when the valve orifice area declines to 1.5 cm^2 or less.

Angiographic imaging of mitral valve stenosis shows characteristic mitral dome formation. This dome formation occurs because the stenotic mitral valve protrudes in a parachute-like shape into the left ventricular cavity. These findings are confirmed by a dome-shaped filling defect on left ventriculography. Clear evidence of dome formation indicates that the valve leaflets are soft and move easily. In cases of severe stenosis, valve excursion deteriorates, and no dome formation is observed. Adhesions on the chordae tendineae below the mitral valve are visible as filling defects. The Sellors classification is generally used to assess the degree of severity.

Echocardiography shows (1) rippling of the mitral valve as seen by M-mode echocardiography, and (2) valvular thickening and commissural adhesions as seen by cross-sectional echocardiography. There may also be findings of dome formation and adhesions in the lower part of the valve. It is important to measure the valve area at this same time.

The Doppler method can be used (1) to observe left ventricular inflow during diastole (approaching from the cardiac apex), (2) to record the narrow cylindrical inflow of blood, (3) to use the continuous-wave Doppler method to measure maximum flow velocity for stenotic blood flow, apply a simplified form of Bernoulli's method [p = $4V^2$ (p, pressure gradient between the left atrium and the left ventricle; V, maximum stenotic flow velocity)], and obtain the mean pressure gradient during diastole in order to calculate the mean mitral valve orifice pressure gradient, and (4) to estimate the area of the mitral valve orifice from stenotic blood flow pressure half-time.

Most patients with mitral stenosis are candidates for open commissurotomy. However, for older patients, valve replacement surgery is indicated in a higher percentage of cases. The key to successful commissurotomy is to thoroughly eliminate valvular stenosis without producing residual regurgitation.

Morphologically characteristic findings for mitral stenosis include (1) thickening and sclerosis of the valve, with adherent thrombi; (2) adhesions of the commissures; (3) thickening, shortening, and adhesions of the chordae tendineae; (4) calcification; (5) the presence of Lambl's excrescences; and (6) stenotic changes in the valve orifice (crescent shape, buttonhole shape). Histologic findings include (1) fibrous changes and hyalinization, (2) neovascularization, (3) calcification, and (4) thrombus formation.

FIG. 26 Resected mitral valve of a 50-year-old woman. At approximately 35 years of age, the patient began to experience dyspnea when climbing stairs. At age 40, she underwent mitral valve commissurotomy, and at age 50 developed heart failure during an episode of upper respiratory infection. The mitral valve was replaced, and aortic valvuloplasty was performed. Thickening, whitening, and opacity of the valve leaflets is shown. Fusion and fibrotic changes are also evident in the chordae tendineae.

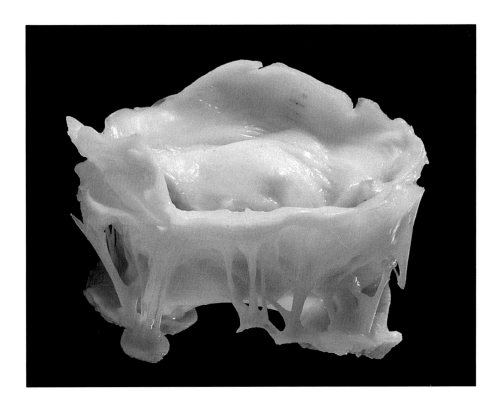

FIG. 27 View of the mitral valve and left atrium of a 67-year-old man after dissection of the posterior wall of the left atrium (cardiac weight 400 g). The patient had been diagnosed with heart disease 4 to 5 years previously. Three months previously, left hemiplegia and dysarthria developed suddenly. Nineteen days previously, the patient became dehydrated. This condition was corrected with treatment, but on admission to the hospital for further evaluation, he suffered a sudden cardiac arrest after eating breakfast and died. Autopsy showed a ball thrombus constricting the mitral valve orifice. The mitral valve leaflets show obvious fibrotic thickening, and commissural fusion and pronounced calcified deposits are visible. The left atrium is enlarged, and the endocardium is whitened due to fibrotic thickening.

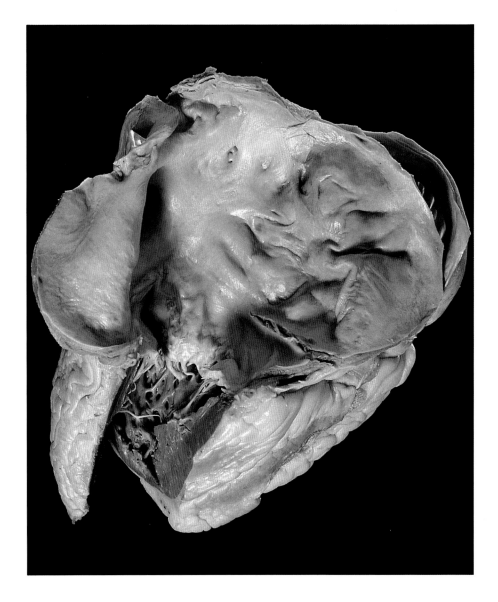

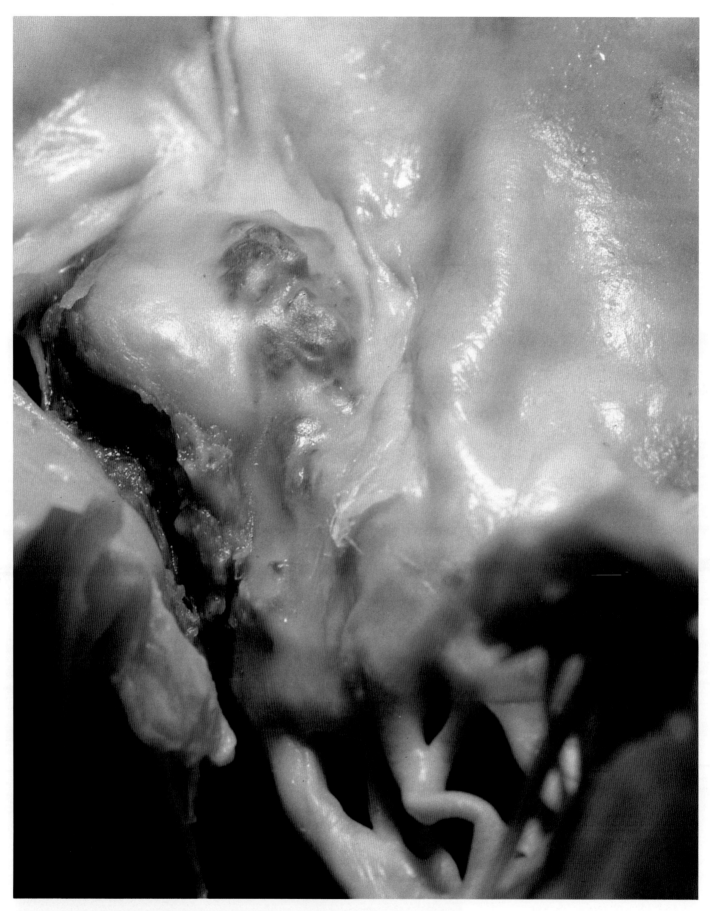

FIG. 28 Enlargement of the anterior commissure and anterior leaflet of the mitral valve in the same case shown in Fig. 27. The anterior leaflet shows pronounced fibrotic thickening; the brown color indicates calcified deposits. Ulceration on the surface of the fused commissures is present, and calcified deposits and adherent thrombi are visible. The chordae tendineae show pronounced fibrotic thickening.

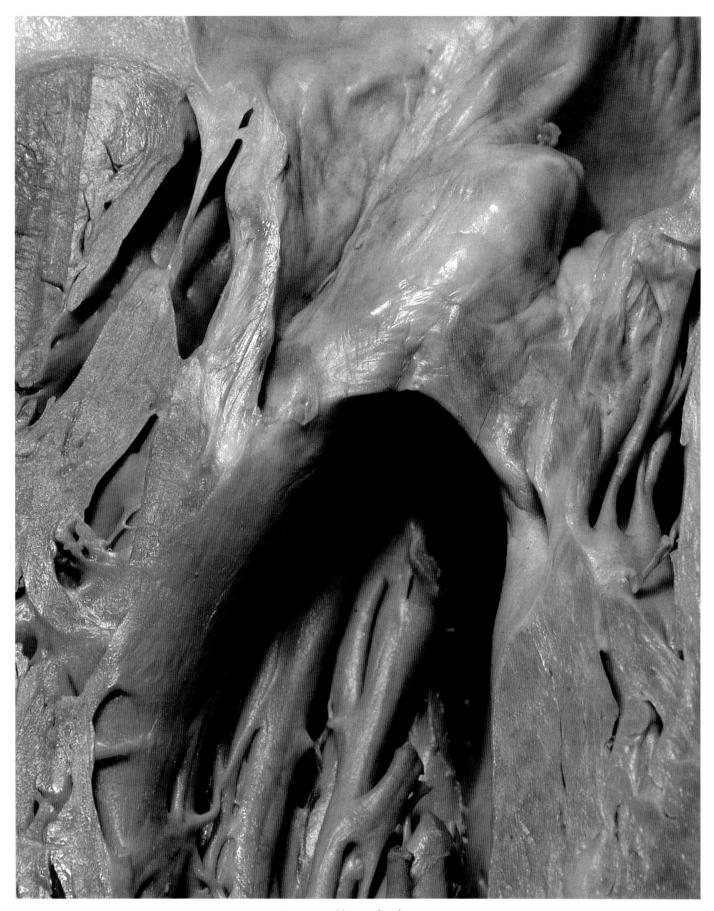

FIG. 29 View of the anterior leaflet of the mitral valve of a 60-year-old man after dissection of the left ventricle (cardiac weight 450 g). The patient was diagnosed with cardiomegaly and atrial fibrillation at age 57. One day before death he suddenly lost strength in both legs, with subsequent cyanosis in the legs. This was followed by multiple thromboemboli and pulmonary edema. The patient was not considered a surgical candidate and subsequently died. Pronounced fibrotic thickening of the valve leaflets is shown. The chordae tendineae are fused and shortened, evidencing fibrotic changes, and the spaces between the chordae tendineae have been eliminated, causing the mitral valve to assume a funnel shape. The valve leaflets can be seen to attach directly to the papillary muscles.

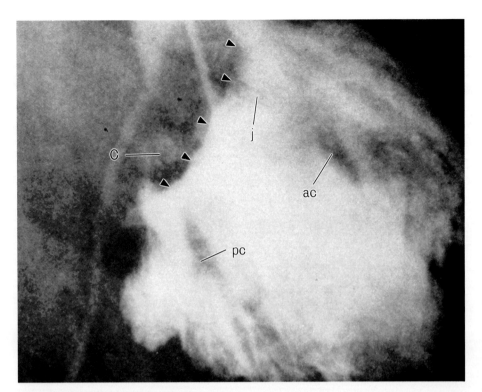

FIG. 30 Left ventriculography, 30-degree right anterior oblique. Mitral valve dome formation (black arrowheads) and filling defects due to subvalvular fusion of the chordae tendineae are evidenced, and a negative jet can be seen from the stenotic valve toward the anterior lateral commissure. The mitral valve shows slight calcification; Sellors grade II stenosis is present. (ac, pc, filling defects; j, jet; C, calcification.)

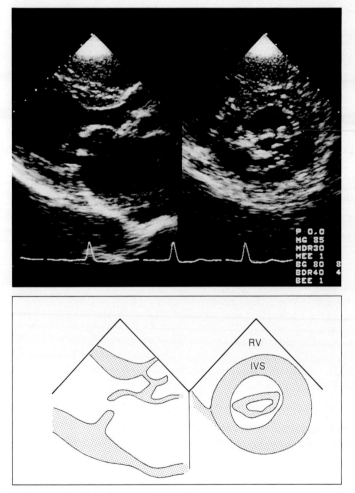

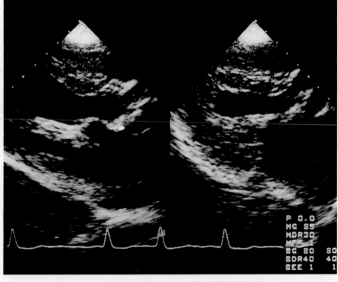

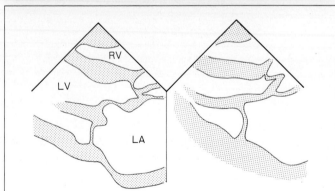

FIG. 31 (Left) Cross-sectional echocardiography on the long axis shows good mobility in the clear zone of the valve, but thickening is evidenced in the rough zone. (Right) Cross-sectional echocardiography on the short axis shows the mitral valve orifice. Adhesions on the posterior commissure are more pronounced than on the anterior commissure. (IVS, intraventricular septum; RV, right ventricle.)

FIG. 32 Cross-sectional echocardiography on the long axis. (Left) Prominent subvalvular lesions on the posterior aspect of the commissure. (Right) Moderate changes in the anterior commissure that are less severe than in the medial commissure (anterior aspect of the commissure). (LA, left atrium; LV, left ventricle; RV, right ventricle.)

FIG. 33 M-mode echocardiography. The anterior leaflet of the mitral valve has lost the bisferient excursion during diastole that is normally seen in healthy subjects. (AML, anterior mitral leaflet; IVS, intraventricular septum; RV, right ventricle.)

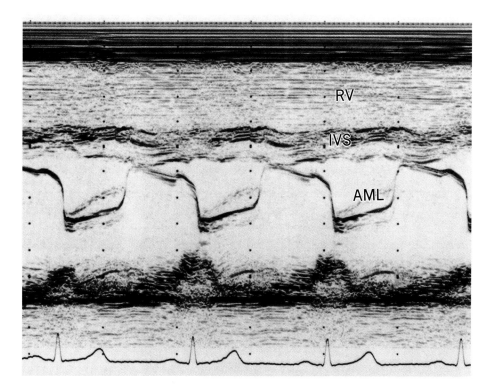

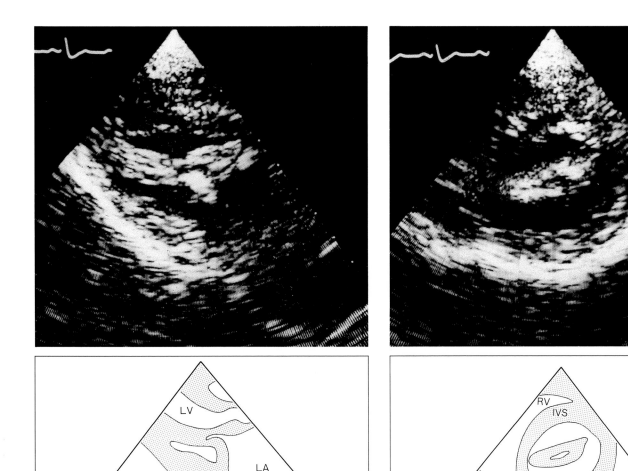

FIG. 34 Severe valve pathology. (Left) Cross-sectional echocardiography on the long axis shows fusion of the valve, chordae tendineae, and papillary muscles. (Right) Cross-sectional echocardiography on the short axis shows fusion and thickening of both the anterior and posterior leaflets and narrowing of the valve orifice. (LA, left atrium; LV, left ventricle; IVS, intraventricular septum; RV, right ventricle.)

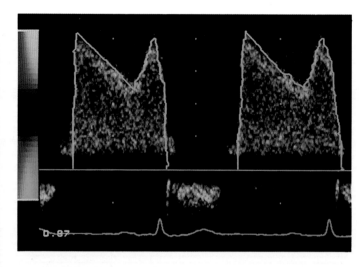

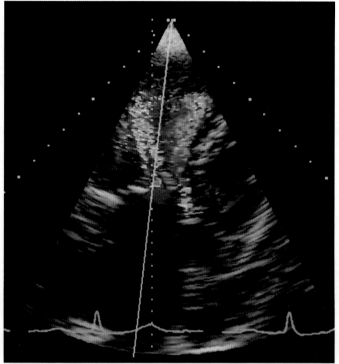

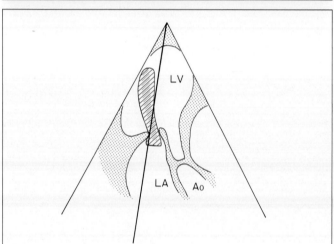

FIG. 35 Doppler imaging. (Left) Cross-section on the long axis, with approach from the cardiac apex. A narrow band-shaped left ventricular inflow is recorded moving from the stenotic mitral valve orifice toward the left ventricular apex. The high velocity of blood flow at the valve orifice produces a reversal due to a turnaliasing phenomenon, recorded in blue, and a mosaic signal. (Right) Continuous-wave Doppler imaging is used to measure maximum inflow velocity. As a method of evaluating the severity of mitral stenosis, this maximum velocity (V) was substituted into a simplified form of Bernoulli's method (p = 4V2) to calculate the mean pressure gradient during diastole, yielding results of 10 mmHg. (Ao, aorta; LA, left atrium; LV, left ventricle.)

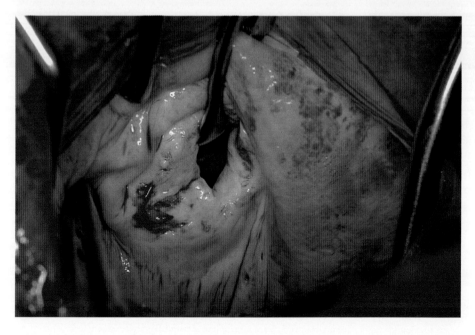

FIG. 36 Intraoperative photograph. The open orifice deviates toward the posterior commissure, and the anterior commissure shows severe fusion. Fresh thrombi can be seen on the valve surface. Commissurotomy was performed in this case.

Mitral Stenosis and Insufficiency (Regurgitation)

Mitral stenosis and insufficiency includes cases involving primarily mitral stenosis, those involving primarily insufficiency (regurgitation), and all intermediate stages; clinical symptoms vary depending on whether stenosis or insufficiency predominates. Almost all cases are complicated by atrial fibrillation.

In this condition, neither stenosis nor insufficiency is necessarily more serious than the other. However, the end stage of rheumatic valvular disease generally involves severe hemodynamic impairment; prognosis is worse than in cases of simple valvular heart disease.

Left ventriculography shows dome formation during diastole and regurgitation during systole. The degree of regurgitation can be evaluated from jet width.

For findings from echocardiography and the Doppler method, refer to the sections, "Mitral Stenosis" and "Mitral insufficiency (Regurgitation)."

Surgical intervention in the form of valvuloplasty is rarely successful in completely eliminating stenosis and insufficiency. Valve replacement is performed in almost all such cases.

Pathologic and morphologic findings include fibrotic changes and shortening of the chordae tendineae, and thickening and involution particularly of the posterior leaflet, which takes on a

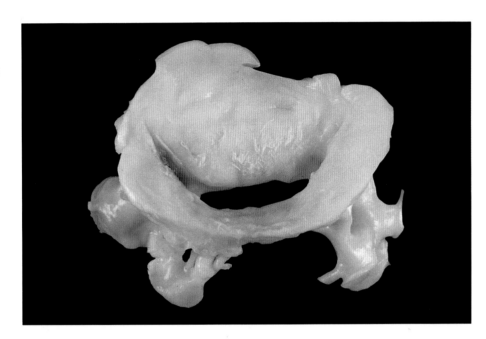

FIG. 37 View from the atrial side of a resected mitral valve from a 49-year-old woman. At age 15 the patient suffered from rheumatic fever. Dyspnea developed at age 23 after delivery of the patient's first child, and valvular heart disease was diagnosed. At age 36, left hemiplegia developed as a result of cerebral infarction, and at age 49, the patient underwent mitral valve replacement, left atrial plication, and tricuspid valvuloplasty. Whitening, loss of transparency, and fibrotic thickening of the valve leaflets is seen. The posterior leaflet is involuted in a fibrous shelf-like shape; the fold-like appearance has been completely lost. The commissures are fused, and severe changes are seen in the chordae tendineae.

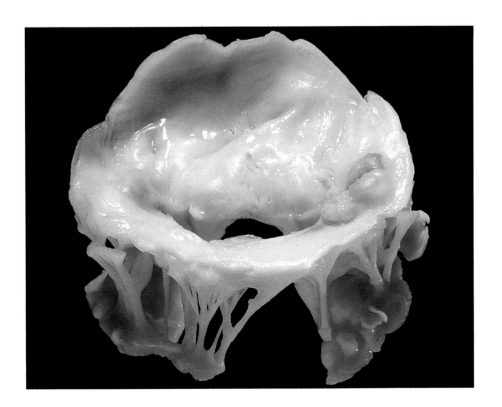

FIG. 38 Resected mitral valve of a 61-year-old woman. The patient was diagnosed with valvular heart disease by her personal physician at approximately 30 years of age. At age 61, she developed heart failure during an upper respiratory infection and underwent mitral valve replacement and annuloplasty of the tricuspid valve. Pronounced fibrotic thickening of the valve leaflets, fusion of the commissures, and brown to black calcified deposits are seen. Pronounced fusion and shortening of the chordae tendineae are also present.

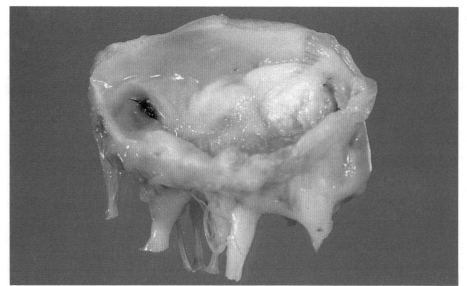

FIG. 39 View from the atrial side of a resected mitral valve of a 58-year-old man. During a physical examination at age 56, a cardiac murmur was detected, followed at age 57, by the detection of arrhythmia and cardiomegaly. At age 58, the patient underwent replacement of the aortic and mitral valves. Fibrotic thickening of the valve leaflets and thickening, fusion, and shortening of the chordae tendineae are shown. The commissures are fused, and obvious calcified deposits are visible. However, some transparency remains in the clear zone.

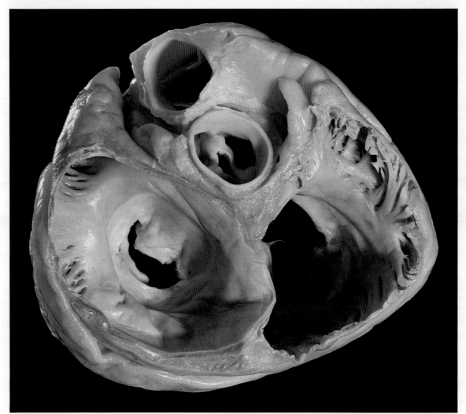

FIG. 40 View of all four valves of a 54-year-old woman after dissection of the left and right atria (cardiac weight 450 g). The patient was diagnosed with valvular heart disease at age 24. One and one-half years before death, the patient developed exertional dyspnea and generalized fatigue. Three months before death, her pulse became irregular, and 2 months before death, she was hospitalized for treatment of heart failure and for further diagnostic evaluation. Although the patient was treated for heart failure and for an arrhythmia, her condition gradually worsened and death ensued. Fibrous thickening of the mitral and aortic valve leaflets, as well as fusion of the commissures, is seen. Enlargement of both the left and right atria is visible.

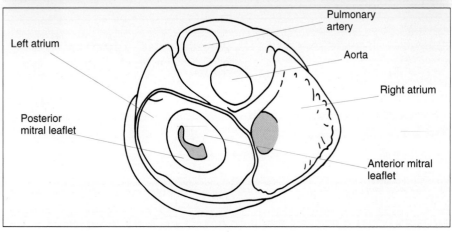

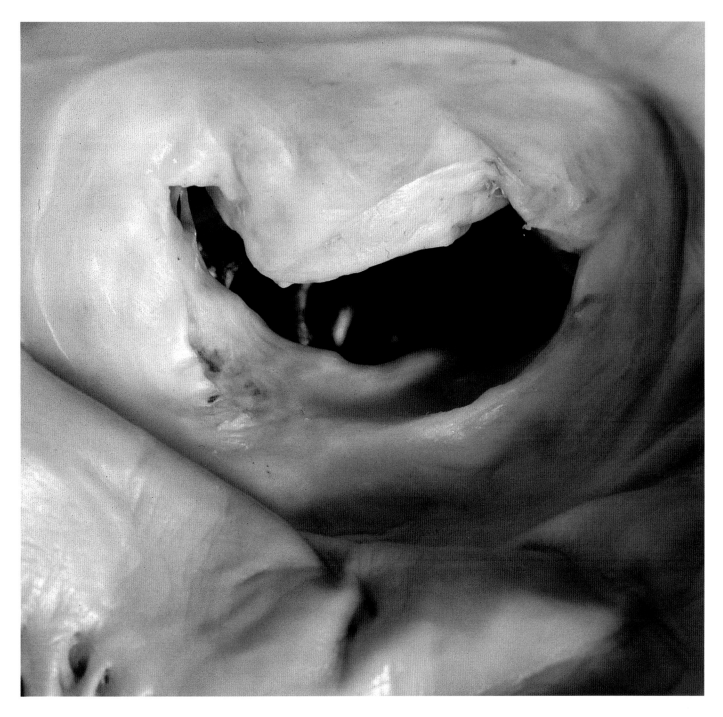

FIG. 41 View from the atrial side of the mitral valve shown in Fig. 40. The valve leaflets show marked fibrotic thickening and fusion of the commissures. The posterior leaflet has lost its fold-like appearance and is involuted, indicating the presence of insufficiency.

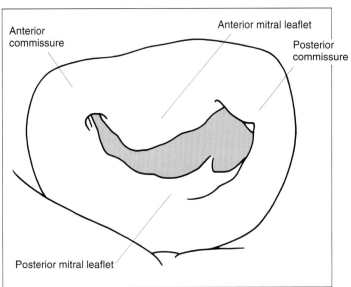

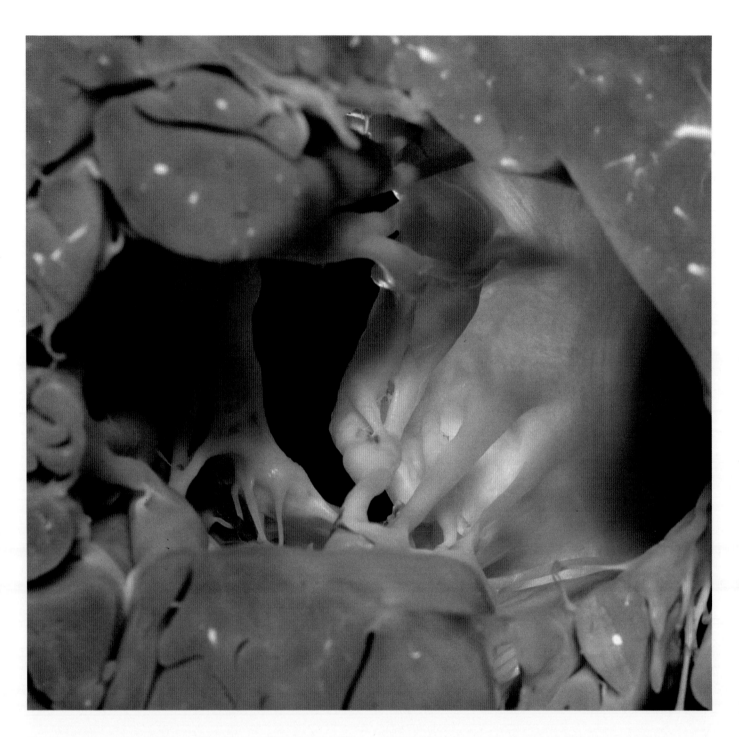

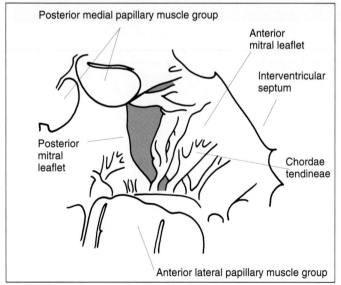

Posterior medial papillary muscle group

Anterior
mitral leaflet

Interventricular
septum

Posterior
mitral
leaflet

Chordae
tendineae

Anterior lateral papillary muscle group

FIG. 42 View from the ventricular side of the mitral valve shown in Fig. 40, showing fusion, shortening, and fibrotic changes in the chordae tendineae.

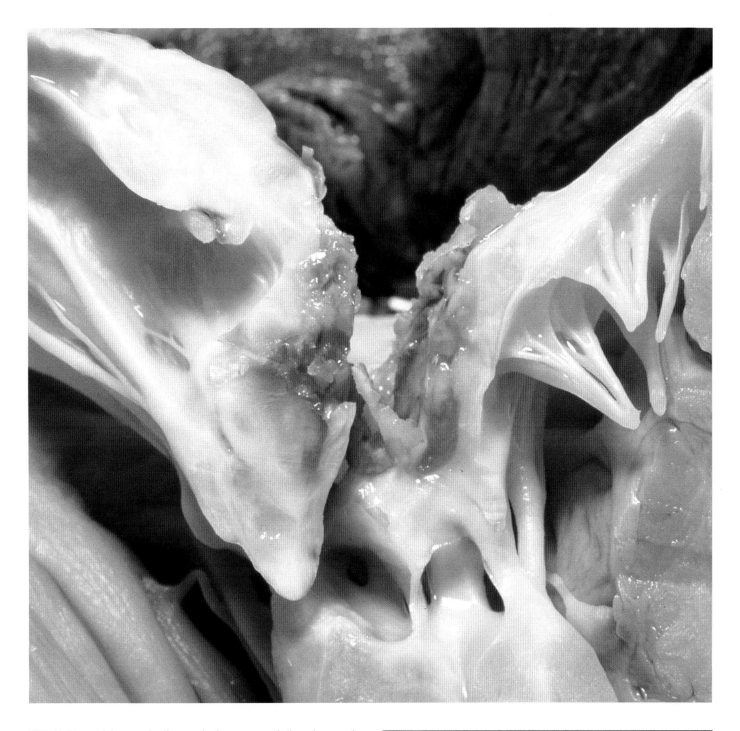

FIG. 43 View of the mitral valve on the long axis, including the mitral valve and the aortic valve (cardiac weight 600 g), of an 80-year-old man. At age 43, combined valvular heart disease was diagnosed. At age 48, the patient underwent an open mitral commissurotomy (OMC). From age 78, dyspnea intensified. Approximately 3 months previously, a cerebral infarction developed in the region of the right posterior cerebral artery. This was followed by exacerbation of heart failure and subsequent death. Marked fibrotic thickening of the valve leaflets is shown. Surface ulceration, calcified deposits, and adherent thrombi are visible. The posterior medial papillary muscle group and the chordae tendineae that attach to it are visible. Fusion, shortening, and fibrotic changes in the chordae tendineae have pulled the papillary muscles into close proximity with the valve leaflets, and the spaces between the chordae tendineae have been eliminated.

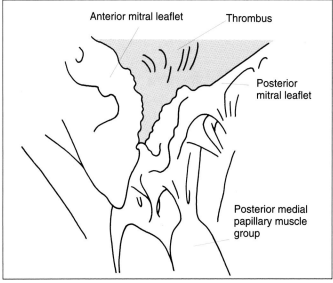

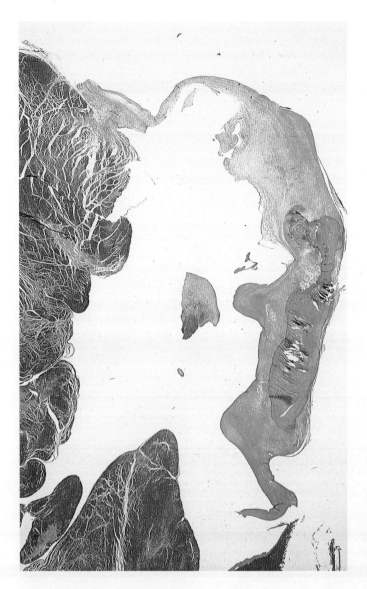

FIG. 44 Tissue section of the posterior leaflet of the mitral valve shown in Fig. 43. The valve leaflet shows marked fibrotic thickening, and calcified deposits are visible. The chordae tendineae also show fibrotic thickening. There is no apparent abnormality at the base of the valve, but there is slight protrusion into the atrium.

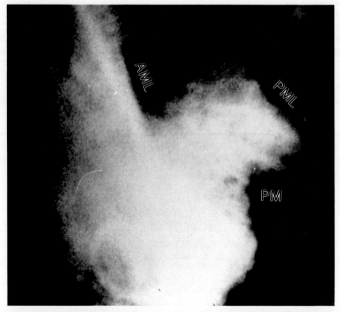

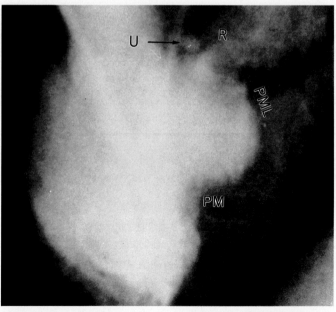

FIG. 45 Angiographic findings indicate hypertrophy and deformation in the subvalvular tissue, particularly the papillary muscles. The posterior leaflet is completely immobile. (Left) During diastole, the anterior leaflet takes on a plate-like shape. (Right) Imaging during systole shows the formation of ulcers (U) on the valve leaflet, and regurgitation (R) can be observed from the connecting areas of both valve leaflets toward the left atrium. The valve leaflets cannot be repaired in such cases; valve replacement surgery is indicated. (AML, anterior valve leaflet; PM, papillary muscle; PML, posterior mitral leaflet.)

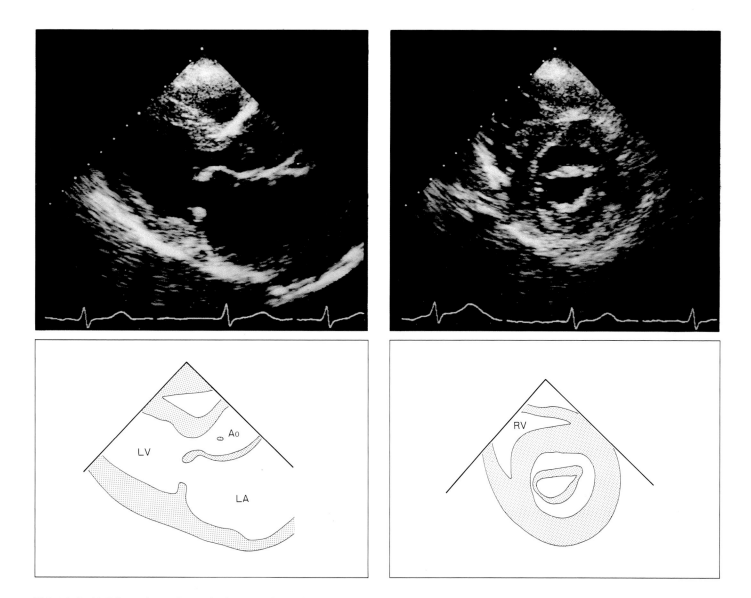

FIG. 46 (Left) Echocardiography on the long axis shows doming of the anterior leaflet of the mitral valve; the posterior leaflet has assumed a wall-like shape with poor mobility. Enlargement of the left atrium is visible. (Right) Echocardiography on the short axis shows that the valve orifice area between the anterior and posterior leaflets of the mitral valve is still adequate. These morphologic findings are not sufficient to confirm mitral insufficiency. (Ao, aorta; LA, left atrium; LV, left ventricle; RV, right ventricle.)

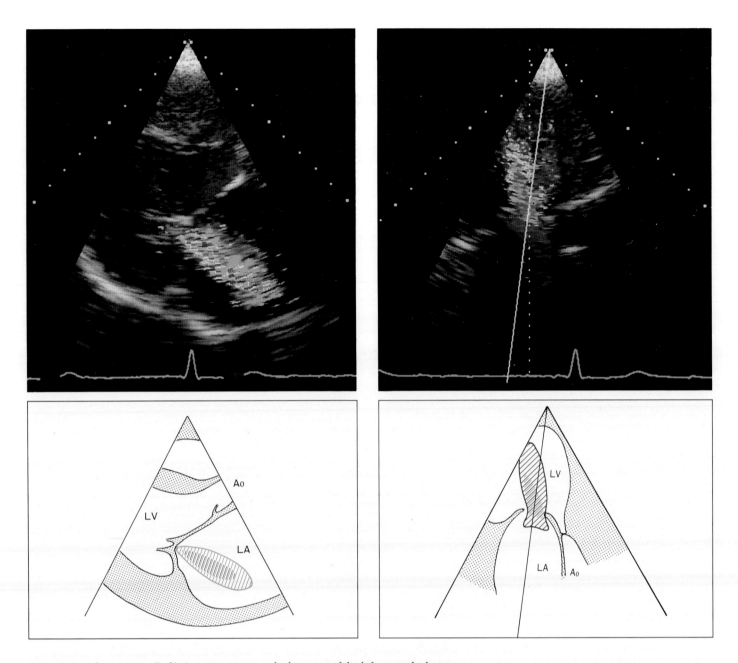

FIG. 47 Doppler imaging. (Left) A cross-section on the long axis of the left ventricle during systole shows a regurgitant jet from the thickened mitral valve into the left atrium. The width of this regurgitant jet indicates moderate regurgitation. (Right) Approaching from the cardiac apex, a cross-section on the long axis of the left ventricle during diastole shows a narrow regurgitant jet from the stenotic mitral valve orifice toward the cardiac apex. Because of the high velocity of flow, the center of the jet shows aliasing (recorded in blue). The peripheral flow is slower and is recorded in red. (Ao, aorta; LA, left atrium; LV, left ventricle.)

Mitral Insufficiency (Regurgitation)

There are six different areas of structural damage that can contribute to mitral insufficiency. These are in the left atrial posterior wall, the mitral valve ring, the mitral valve leaflets, the chordae tendineae, the papillary muscles, and the left ventricular wall. In cases of rheumatic mitral insufficiency, the valve orifice is known to close insufficiently during systole. Valve thickening and adhesions on the commissures are major contributing factors. Regurgitation produces enlargement of the left atrium and left ventricle. Enlargement of the mitral valve ring and disturbance of the papillary muscle structures can also exacerbate valvular insufficiency.

When using diagnostic angiography, the degree of mitral insufficiency can be judged from the width and extent of the jet that is directed toward the left atrium during left ventricular systole, and from the concentration of the contrast agent in the left atrium. When the jet is narrow, little regurgitation is present; as regurgitation increases, the jet widens. In severe regurgitation, the contrast agent extends from the entire valve orifice toward the left ventricle. A four-stage scale is used for evaluation: mild, moderate, severe, and "very severe."

Echocardiography shows valvular thickening, shearing, and gaps at the contact surfaces between the anterior and posterior leaflets, and enlargement of the mitral valve ring.

Using the Doppler method with a parasternal and apical approach, structures can be examined stereoscopically from the mitral valve orifice throughout the entire left atrium. First, regurgitant signal is recorded during systole when blood is ejected from the mitral valve orifice into the left atrium. Second, the regurgitant area for the maximum recorded cross-section as measured by the regurgitant signal is used as an indicator, and regurgitation is classified on a four-stage scale. Third, the site of regurgitation can be identified from the regurgitation location as recorded in cross-section along the short axis of the mitral valve orifice. In this case, irregular blood flow can be observed even when the site of regurgitation is on the left ventricular side. This signal can help to identify the site of regurgitation.

Severe structural changes are common in insufficiency that results from rheumatic valvular disease. These patients are generally candidates for surgical intervention in the form of valve replacement. However, valvuloplasty is sometimes performed in cases of mild stenotic lesions.

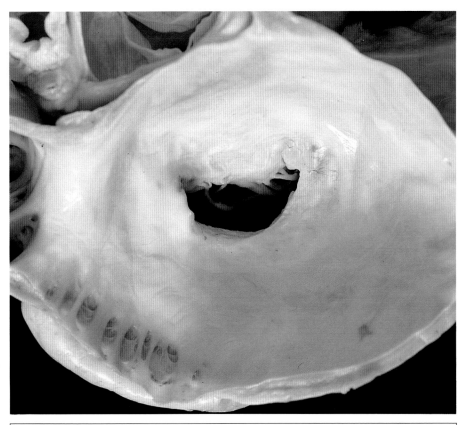

FIG. 48 View of the mitral valve from the atrial side of an 81-year-old man after dissection of the left atrium (cardiac weight 650 g). At age 63, the patient was diagnosed with atrial fibrillation. From age 77, he developed exertional dyspnea, and at age 78 was diagnosed with valvular heart disease. At age 81, the patient died of complications of pneumonia. Obvious fibrotic thickening of the mitral valve leaflets, adhesions on the commissures, and calcified deposits on the anterior commissure are shown. The posterior leaflet is involuted and has a shelf-like appearance.

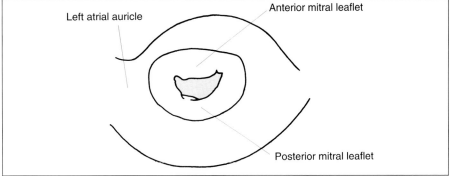

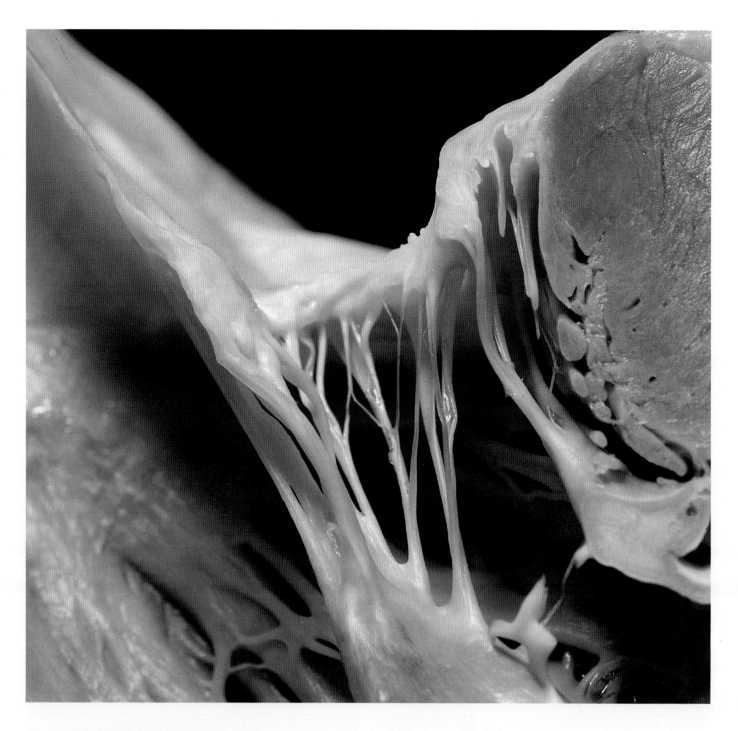

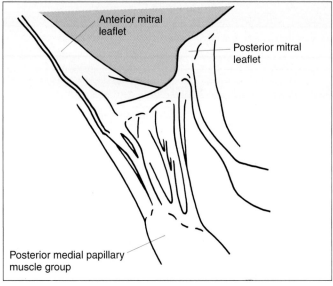

Anterior mitral leaflet

Posterior mitral leaflet

Posterior medial papillary muscle group

FIG. 49 The mitral valve seen along the long axis, including the mitral valve and the aortic valve, of the same case in discussed in Fig. 48. The valve leaflets show fibrotic thickening, and the posterior leaflet has a shelf-like appearance. The posterior medial papillary muscle group and attached chordae tendineae are visible; the chordae tendineae show mild fibrotic changes and adhesions.

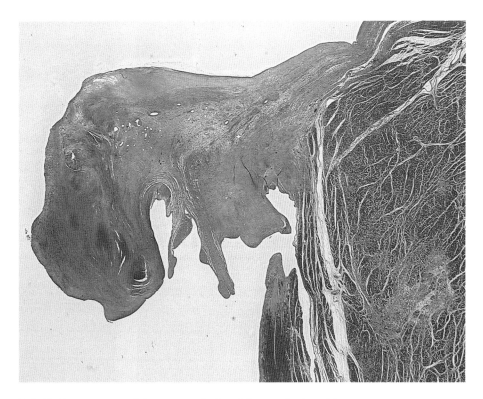

FIG. 50 Tissue section of the posterior leaflet of the mitral valve of the case discussed in Fig. 48. The valve leaflet shows pronounced fibrotic thickening, and an increase in microvascularization is evident. There is also obvious thickening of the chordae tendinea.

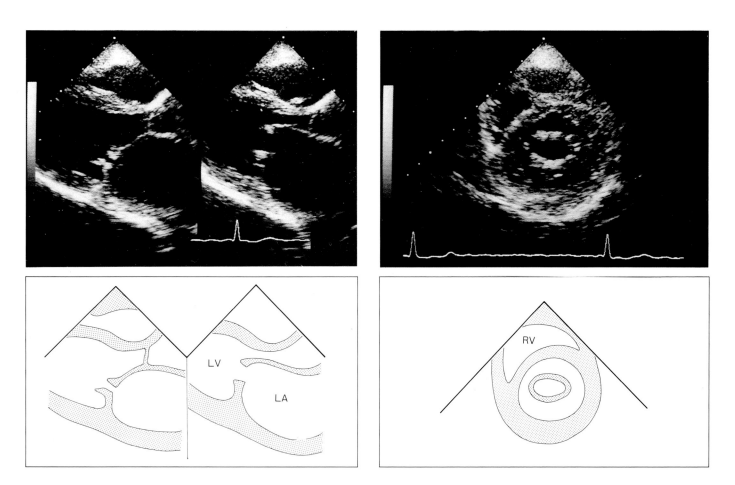

FIG. 51 (Left) Cross-sectional echocardiography on the long axis shows thickening in the rough zone. Because of enlargement of the valve ring, the image on the left, during systole, shows spaces between the anterior and posterior leaflets. (Right) Cross-sectional echocardiography along the short axis shows wide opening of the mitral valve orifice and little fusion of the commissures. (LA, left atrium; LV, left ventricle; RV, right ventricle.)

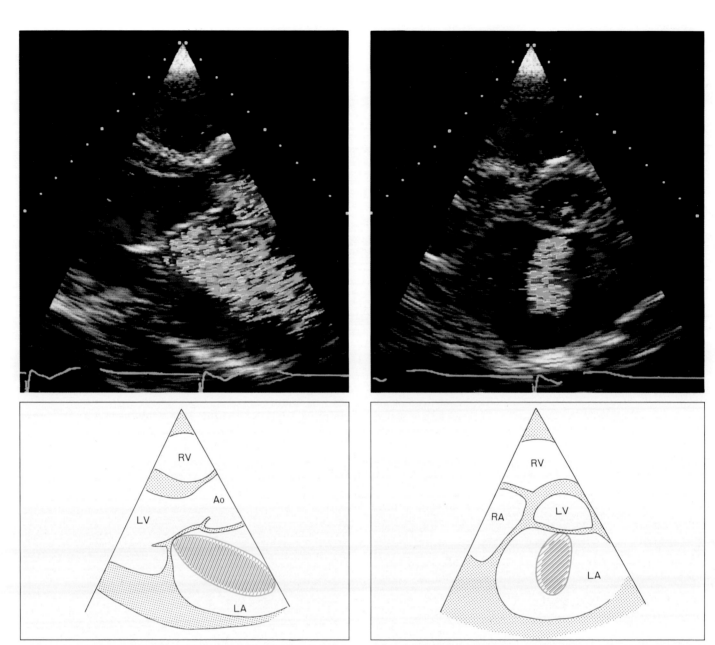

FIG. 52 Two-dimensional Doppler angiography. (Left) A cross-section on the long axis of the left ventricle records a broad jet-shaped regurgitant signal from the mitral valve orifice into the atrium. (Right) A cross-sectional view on the short axis of the left ventricle records an ellipse-shaped regurgitant signal from the center of the mitral valve orifice. Because of the width of the regurgitant signal, severe regurgitation is judged to be present. (Ao, aorta; LA, left atrium; LV, left ventricle; RA, right atrium; RV, right ventricle.)

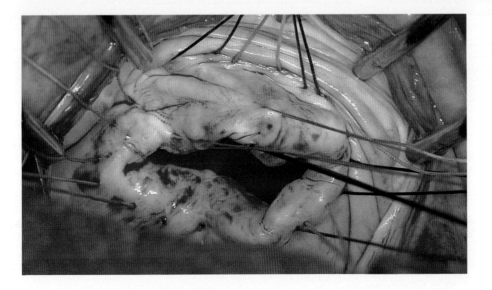

FIG. 53 Intraoperative photograph showing thickening of the valve leaflets and slight fusion of the commissures. Hemodynamically, this is a case of pure mitral insufficiency. The sutures are placed around the entire perimeter of the valve ring for ring annuloplasty.

Giant Left Atrium

A giant left atrium accompanying mitral valvular disease frequently persists even after surgery as a major anomaly, and often complicates postoperative circulatory and respiratory management. Although the mechanism of injury is not fully understood, compression of the surrounding organs due to a giant left atrium is an extremely serious problem in surgical intervention.

Of the forms of compression injury resulting from enlargement of the left atrium, three pathophysiologic mechanisms in particular can have a pronounced effect on the postoperative course. These are (1) impingement on the posterior wall of the left ventricle from progressive enlargement of the left atrium downwards, (2) impingement on the left bronchial tube due to expansion to the left and upwards, and (3) impingement on the central and lower lobes of the right lung from expansion to the right. In the first, the impinged basal aspect of the posterior left ventricle shows paradoxical motion. After valve replace-

ment surgery, nonphysiologic blood flow into the left atrium will be observed; this can be a factor in reduced postoperative cardiac function. The latter two conditions cause atelectasis or a reduction in lung capacity from their respective positions, and in particular can be major causes of postoperative respiratory failure.

Echocardiography may show that the left atrium has caused the basal aspect of the posterior left ventricle to encroach on the anterior chest wall. For findings from the Doppler method, see the sections "Stenosis" and "Mitral Insufficiency (Regurgitation)."

Because this condition can produce life-threatening postoperative compression injury on the surrounding organs, left atrial plication is also performed when mitral valve surgery is undertaken.

Morphologic findings in addition to a giant left atrium include (1) endocardial thickening in the left atrium, (2) thrombi on the left atrial wall, and (3) organization of thrombi on the wall.

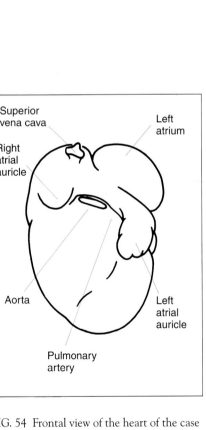

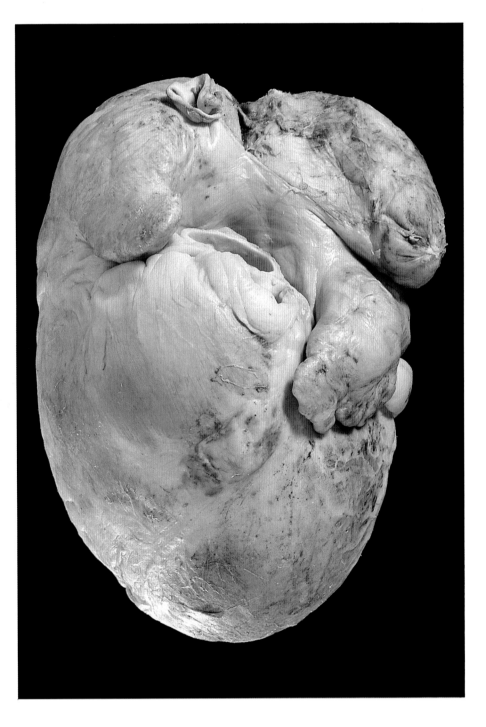

FIG. 54 Frontal view of the heart of the case discussed in Fig. 48. Cardiac weight is 650 g. Pronounced hypertrophy and dilation is present. Enlargement of the left atrium is particularly marked, with thinning of the walls. The left atrial dilation gives the appearance of two left atrial auricles.

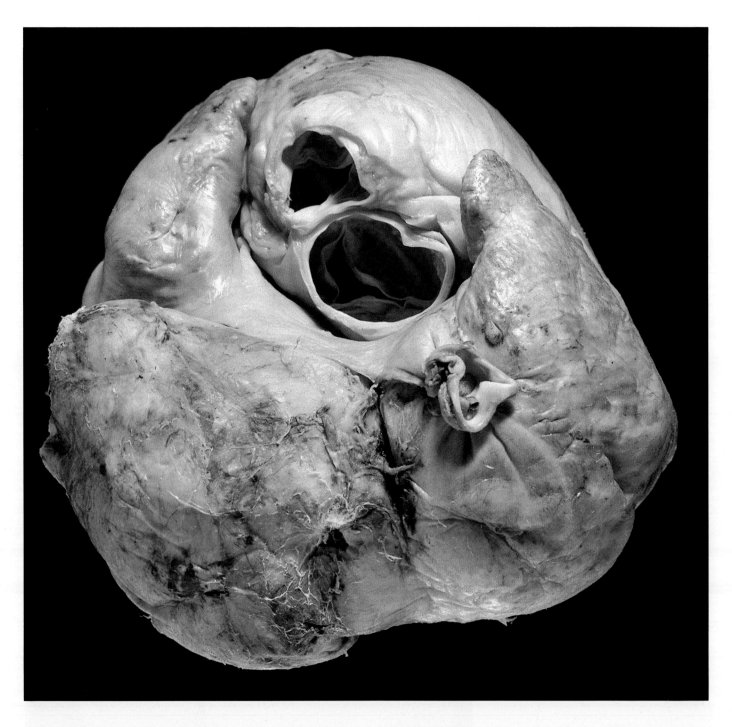

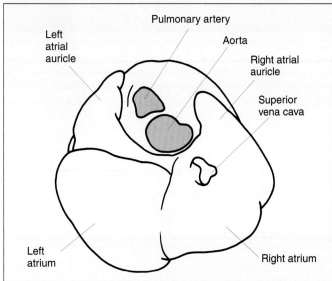

FIG. 55 Cephalad view of the heart from the case discussed in Fig. 48. Marked dilation of the left and right atria is present; dilation of the left atrium is particularly pronounced.

Labels on diagram: Pulmonary artery, Left atrial auricle, Aorta, Right atrial auricle, Superior vena cava, Left atrium, Right atrium

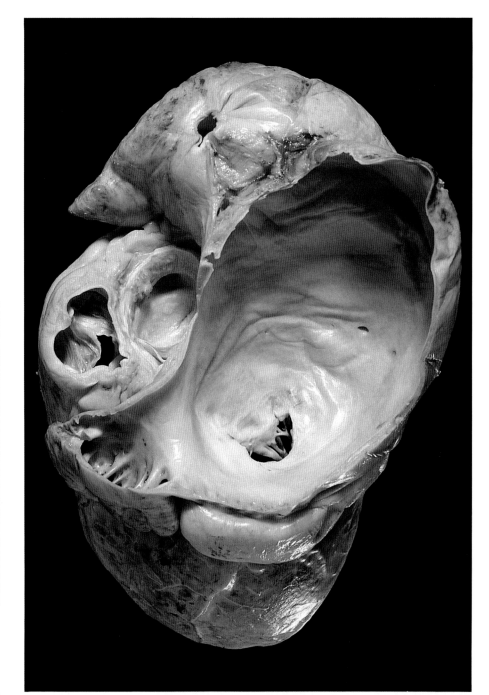

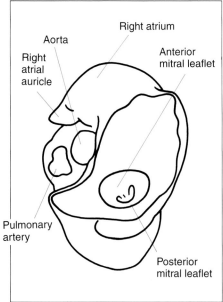

FIG. 56 View of the mitral valve and left atrial lumen after dissection of the anterior and left walls of the left atrium (same case as in Fig. 48). The mitral valve shows fibrotic thickening of the valve leaflets, there are adhesions on the commissures, and the posterior leaflet is involuted. The left atrium is markedly dilated, with thinning of the walls.

FIG. 57 Plain chest radiograph. Pronounced enlargement in the area of the left atrial appendage is present, and atelectasis can be observed in the left lower lung field.

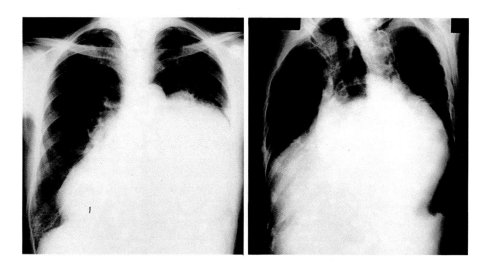

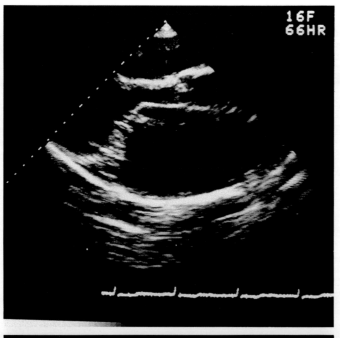

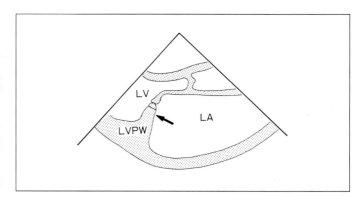

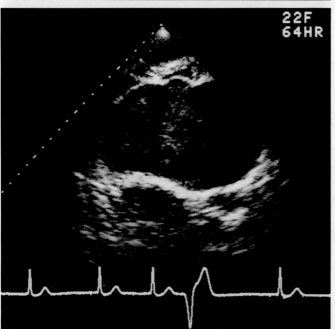

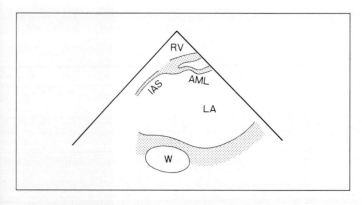

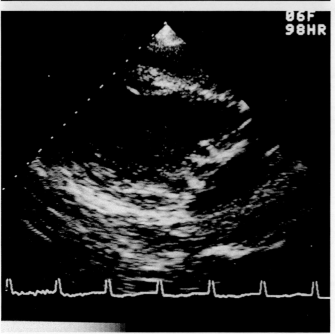

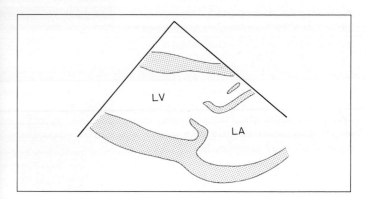

FIG. 58 Echocardiography. (Top) Preoperative. Enlarged left atrium in contact with the dorsal aspect of the posterior wall of the left ventricle. The arrow indicates, not the posterior leaflet of the mitral valve, but the posterior wall of the left ventricle. (Middle) Preoperative. Giant left atrium on both sides of the vertebra. The interatrial septum impinges into the left atrium. (Bottom) Postoperative. The findings observed before surgery have been eliminated. The mitral valve has been replaced with a tissue valve. (AML, anterior mitral leaflet; IAS, interatrial septum; LA, left atrium; LV, left ventricle; LVPW, left ventricular posterior wall; RV, right ventricle; W, vertebra.)

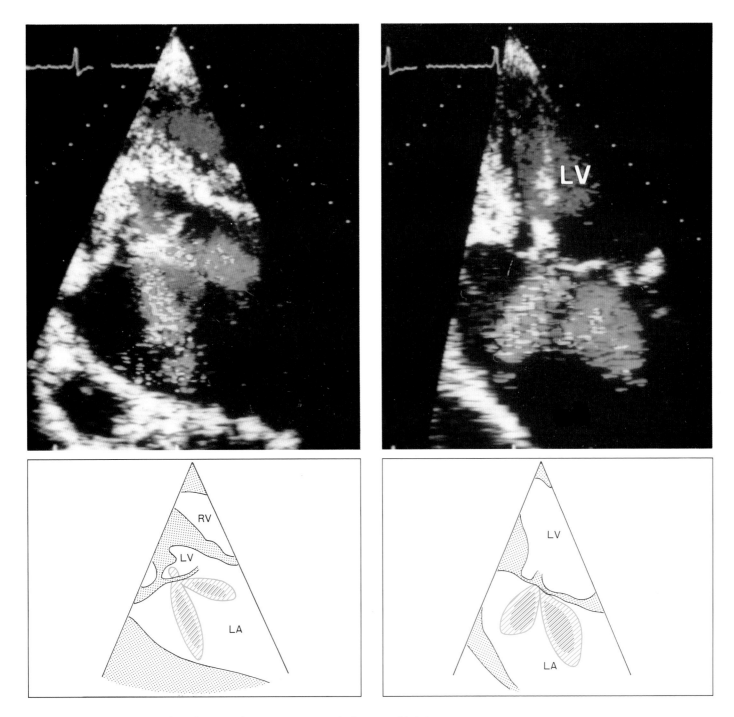

FIG. 59 Doppler imaging. (Left) Left ventricular cross-section on the long axis (slightly lateral to medial). Bifurcated jet-shaped regurgitant signal from the mitral valve orifice to the left atrial lumen is seen. The width of the regurgitant signal indicates severe regurgitation. (LA, left atrium; LV, left ventricle; RV, right ventricle.)

Left Atrial Thrombus

Left atrial thrombus is a complication of mitral stenosis. Its incidence is increased in proportion to the enlargement of the left atrium. Left atrial thrombus occurs most commonly within the left atrial auricle, sometimes forming a polyp-shaped protuberance. Mural thrombus formation frequently accompanies calcification. Rarely, ball thrombus formation is also observed; these ball thrombi are believed to occlude the opening of the pulmonary artery. The presence of left atrial thrombus is generally complicated by atrial fibrillation.

Mural Thrombus

Diagnostic imaging of mural thrombi within the left atrium is difficult. When the thrombi are very large, they can be seen as filling defects on pulmonary angiography, but thrombi that are only weakly attached cannot be diagnosed by this method. Thrombi in the left atrial auricle may show a smoke-like image with left coronary angiography.

A careful search of the left atrial auricle for thrombi is required on echocardiography. Echocardiographic images may show mural thrombi as abnormal structures taking on a tumor-like appearance within the left atrium.

The presence of mural thrombi alone does not make a patient a candidate for surgical intervention, but mobile thrombi may require early surgery. It is quite difficult to remove a mural thrombus completely by excision of the thrombus alone, so scraping with excision of the pseudoendothelium is also performed.

Pathologic and morphologic findings show (1) left atrial endothelial thickening (mural thrombus organization) and (2) calcification of the left atrial wall.

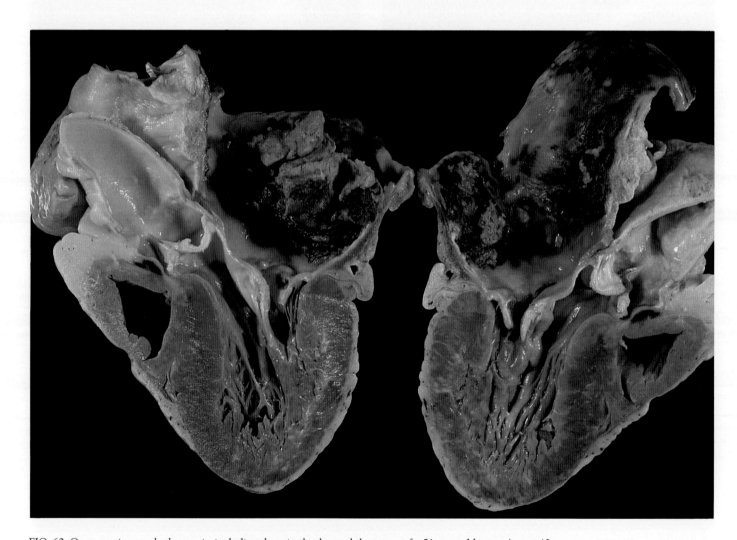

FIG. 60 Cross-section on the long axis, including the mitral valve and the aorta, of a 51-year-old man. At age 40, the patient suddenly developed paralysis of the right upper extremity, and heart disease was diagnosed. At age 45, exertional dyspnea appeared. Five months before death, exertional dyspnea worsened. Two months before death, left visual anomalies developed, and the patient was admitted to the hospital for further diagnostic testing. While in the hospital, multiple thromboemboli occurred and the patient died. Pronounced enlargement of the left atrium is shown; a large mural thrombus is visible. Left ventricular hypertrophy is present, and diffuse fibrotic changes are visible. The mitral valve leaflets show fibrotic thickening accompanied by fusion of the chordae tendineae, and there are indications of funnel-shaped stenosis. The aortic valve also shows fibrotic thickening.

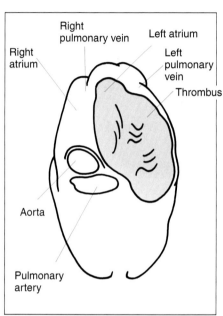

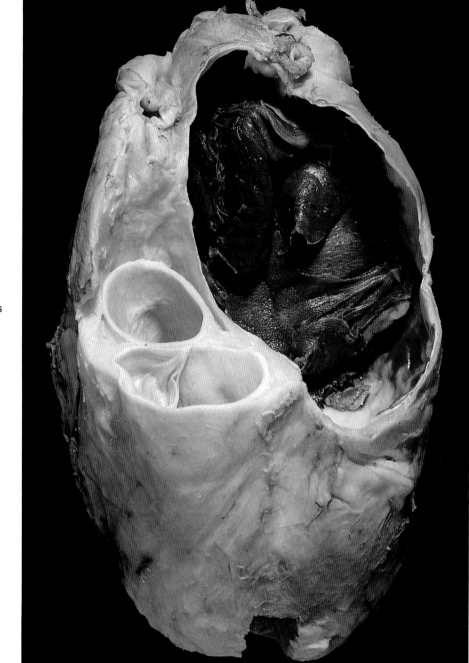

FIG. 61 View of a mural thrombus in the left atrium of an 80-year-old man after dissection of the left anterior and left lateral walls (cardiac weight 600 g). At age 43, the patient was diagnosed with combined valvular heart disease. At age 48, he underwent an open mitral commissurotomy (OMC). Dyspnea worsened from age 78. Approximately 3 months before death, cerebral infarction developed in the region of the right posterior cerebral artery, after which heart failure worsened and death ensued. A large thrombus from the interatrial septum to the posterior wall of the left atrium is shown. Perfusion obstruction of the pulmonary artery is not present.

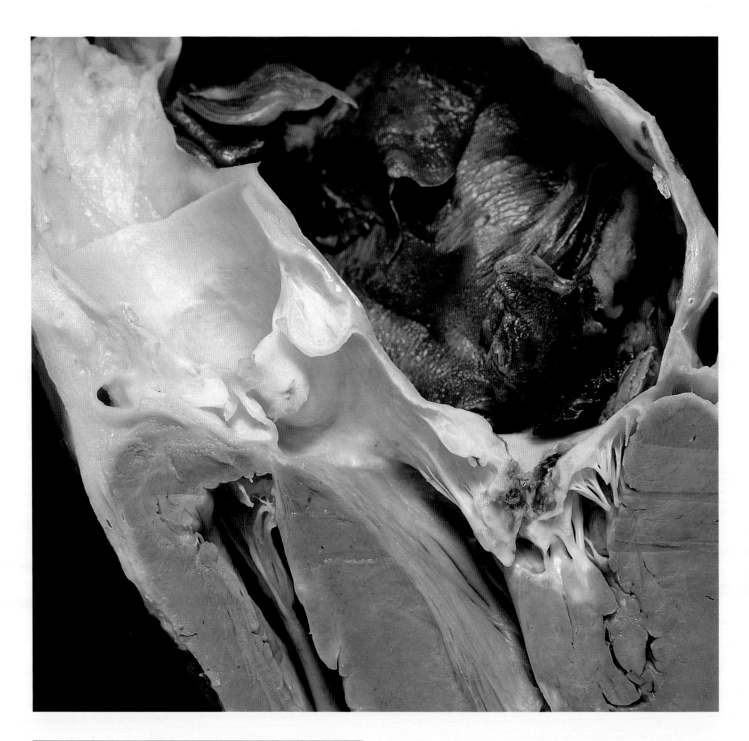

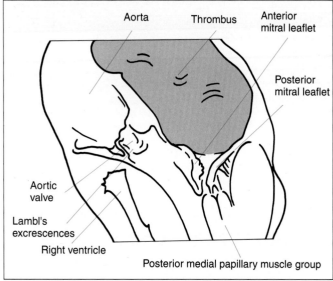

Aorta   Thrombus   Anterior
mitral leaflet

Posterior
mitral leaflet

Aortic
valve

Lambl's
excrescences

Right ventricle

Posterior medial papillary muscle group

FIG. 62 Cross-section of the long axis, including both the mitral and aortic valves, of the case discussed in Fig. 61, showing pronounced fibrotic thickening of the mitral valve, calcified deposits, superficial ulceration, and thrombi. The chordae tendineae are fused, shortened, and fibrotic, and the valve orifice displays a funnel shape. A large mural thrombus is visible within the enlarged left aorta. There are Lambl's excrescences (projections) attached to the aortic noncoronary cusp.

FIG. 65 Enhanced CT scan showing left atrial thrombus (arrow) and calcification of the mitral valve (white triangle). (Ao, aorta; LA, left atrium; PA, pulmonary artery; RA, right atrium; SVC, superior vena cava.)

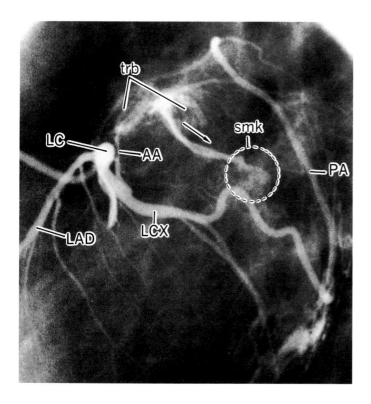

FIG. 63 Angiography of the left coronary artery, 60-degree left anterior oblique. From the bifurcation of the anterior atrial branch, the mural thrombus in the auricle of the left atrium demonstrates blushing (trb). From this point, the contrast agent diffuses to the superior posterior wall of the auricle, where it appears as a smoky haze, flows into the left atrium, and vanishes (arrow). (AA, anterior atrial branch; smk, smoke-like image; LC, left coronary artery; LAD, left anterior descending branch; LCX, left circumflex coronary artery; PA, posterior atrial branch.)

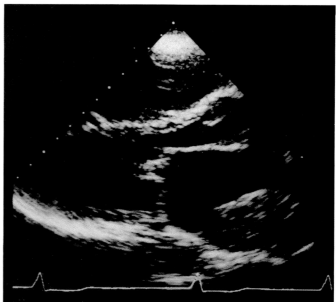

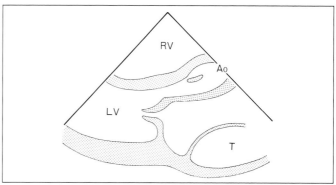

FIG. 64 Cross-sectional echocardiography on the long axis. Rheumatic mitral valvular disease is complicated by thrombi diffusely adherent to the posterior wall of the left atrium. (Ao, aorta; LV, left ventricle; RV, right ventricle; T, thrombus.)

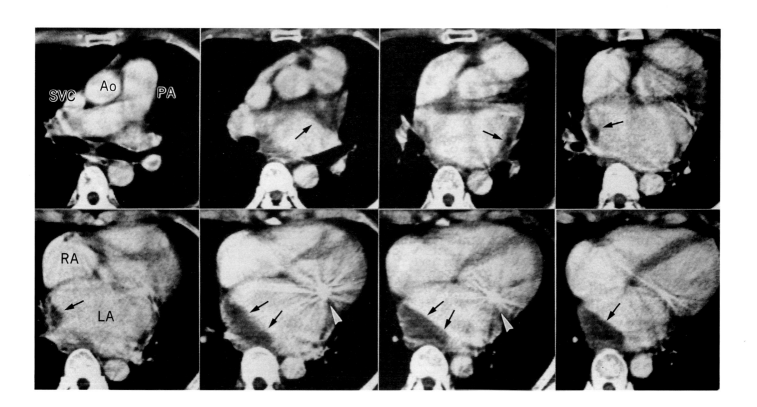

Ball Thrombus

On transpulmonary cineangiography, large ball thrombi are visible as spherical filling defects that move back and forth within the left atrium. Echocardiography shows these ball thrombi as abnormal tumor-shaped structures within the left atrium. It is necessary to search very carefully for thrombi within the auricle of the left atrium.

Ball-thrombus emboli can be life threatening; emergency surgery is indicated immediately on discovery.

Characteristic pathologic and morphologic findings include (1) the presence of mixed thrombi, (2) adherence to the auricle or valve, and (3) fibrin stripes (lines of Zahn).

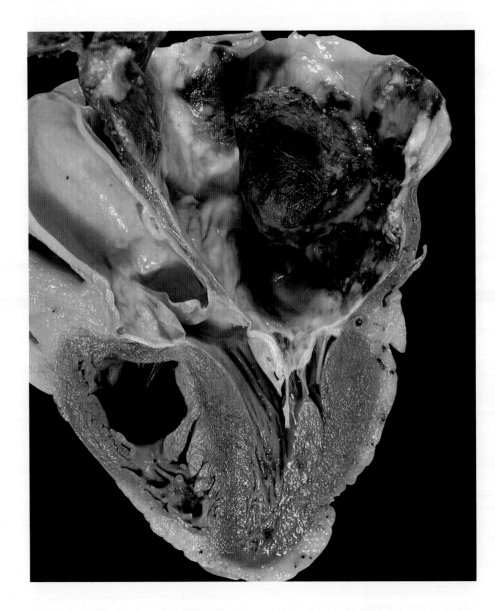

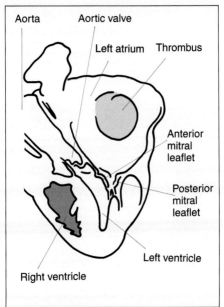

FIG. 66 Cross-section on the long axis, including the aortic valve and the mitral valve (cardiac weight 470 g) of a 72-year-old woman. At age 41, abnormal ECG findings were detected. The patient was diagnosed with mitral stenosis, enlargement of the left atrium, and left atrial thrombus. There was no worsening of subjective symptoms, and the patient remained at NYHA class II, but at age 72, she developed chest pains that progressed to cardiac arrest and death ensued. Enlargement of the left atrium and narrowing of the left ventricle is shown. Pronounced calcification and fibrotic thickening of the mitral valve are present, and the chordae tendineae are thickened and shortened. Ball thrombi are visible within the enlarged left atrium, and some have adhered to the left atrial wall. The atrial endocardium shows endocardial thickening and fresh thrombus formation as a result of organization of the mural thrombi.

FIG. 67 View of the mitral valve and ball thrombus of the case discussed in Fig. 66. Fibrin and red blood corpuscles produce a red-brown color on the surface of the ball thrombus. The white areas indicate organization. The mitral valve also shows adhesion of the commissures.

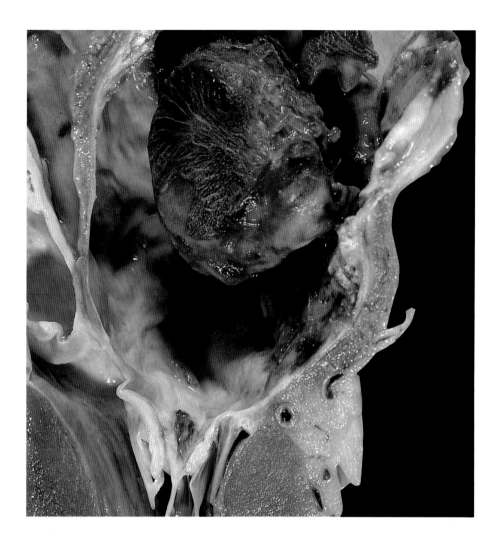

FIG. 68 Cross-section of the ball thrombus shown in Fig. 66. The interior of the ball thrombus is white, and consists primarily of fibrin and platelets. Red thrombi are present laterally, making this a mixed thrombus. The thrombus is contiguous with a mural thrombus in the left atrium.

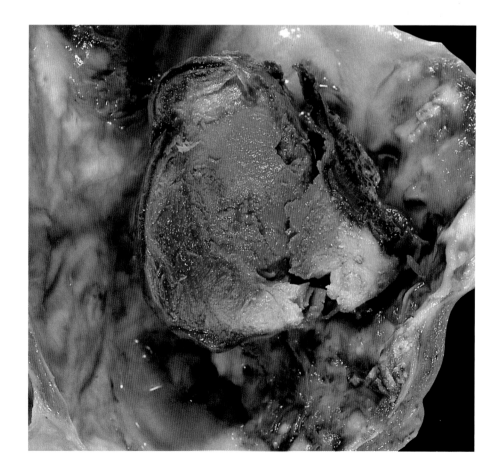

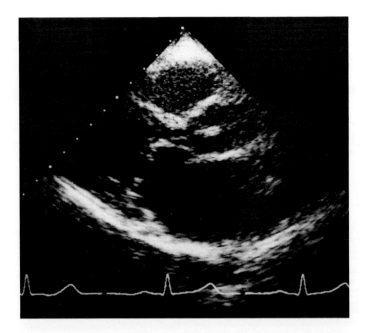
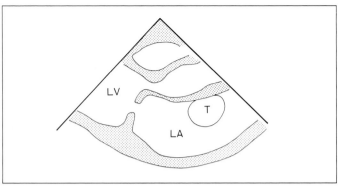

FIG. 69 Cross-sectional echocardiography on the long axis, showing a ball thrombus on the anterior wall of the left atrium. It is rare to find left atrial thrombi on the anterior wall of the left atrium; such findings must be carefully distinguished from ulcers. When the thrombus is only narrowly attached, careful attention should be paid to the possibility of embolism formation. (LA, left atrium; LV, left ventricle; T, thrombus.)

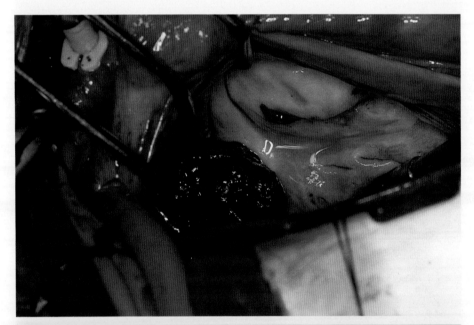

FIG. 70 Intraoperative photograph. Following a cerebral embolism, echocardiography showed the presence of a ball thrombus, and emergency surgery was performed. Dissection of the left atrium revealed a thrombus the size of the tip of a thumb (top figure). This thrombus was removed, and commissurotomy and closure of the left auricle were performed.

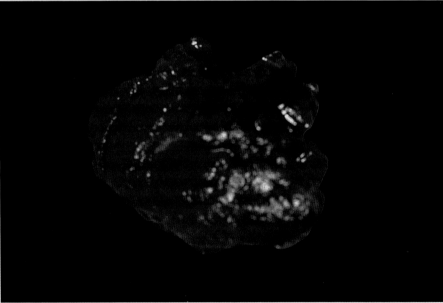

Mitral Valve Prolapse

Mitral valve prolapse is defined as a deviation of the mitral valve from its normal position toward the left atrium. This produces shearing at the valve contact surfaces and gives rise to mitral insufficiency.

Cases of mitral valve prolapse can be divided into those in which the etiology is completely unknown, and those in which prolapse of the mitral valve accompanies obvious heart disease and connective tissue disease. The former is termed *idiopathic mitral valve prolapse,* and the latter *secondary mitral valve prolapse.* Forms of heart disease that can cause secondary mitral valve prolapse include ostium secundum interatrial septal defect, hypertrophic obstructive cardiomyopathy, coronary artery disease, and diseases that produce deformation of the left ventricle. Connective tissue diseases include Marfan syndrome, Ehlers-Danlos syndrome, and Hurler syndrome.

Characteristic morphology in mitral valve prolapse ranges from near-normal structures to severe pathophysiology. Cross-sectional echocardiography has proved the most useful tool for diagnosis of this condition.

Mitral valve prolapse becomes progressively more serious with aging, and mitral insufficiency worsens, giving rise to heart failure. In some cases, drug therapy proves inadequate and surgical intervention is required.

Complications include ruptured chordae tendineae and infectious endocarditis. Histopathologic studies show myxomatous changes at the site of the lesion. Within the valvular tissue, fusion and degeneration of the collagen fibers in the pars fibrosa are considered major factors in some theories.

Mitral Valve Prolapse Without Ruptured Chordae

Left ventriculography shows protrusion of the anterior leaflet or the posterior leaflet into the left atrium during systole. These findings can be observed on 30-degree right anterior oblique or 60-degree left anterior oblique (hepatoclavicular) views. Severe prolapse causes regurgitation.

Echocardiographic findings are diagnostic if shearing is detected at the contact surfaces of the mitral valve and if the mitral valve is observed to deviate toward the left atrium from the normal position of the mitral annulus.

The Doppler method shows a regurgitant jet moving in the opposite direction from the prolapsed valve. However, in cases of prolapse of the posterior leaflet with medial or lateral scalloping, the regurgitant jet shifts toward the opposite commissure, as if crossing the mitral valve orifice. The severity of regurgitation is normally assessed by the usual criteria for mitral insufficiency. But because regurgitation occurs along the left atrial wall in many cases, there is a tendency to underestimate the severity of regurgitation.

Surgical intervention basically involves valvuloplasty that combines annular plication and the shortening of the elongated chordae tendineae. Prognosis for valvuloplasty is poor in cases in which extensive valvular prolapse is present.

Characteristic histopathologic findings include (1) thickening of the valve leaflets, (2) nonfibrotic myxomatous changes, (3) soft transparent appearance, (4) similar findings in the chordae tendineae (up to the point of rupture), (5) histologic findings of myxomatous degeneration, and (6) tearing of the connective tissue layer.

FIG. 71 View from the atrial side of a resected mitral valve of a 45-year-old woman. Valvular disease was diagnosed at age 42. At age 44, the patient underwent cardiac catheterization at another hospital; results indicated that she was not a candidate for surgery at that time. At age 54, both the mitral and tricuspid valves were replaced. A white opacity on the perimeter of the valve leaflets is shown. The leaflets are thickened, but the valve base is thin and remains transparent. The chordae tendineae are whitened, opaque, and fused.

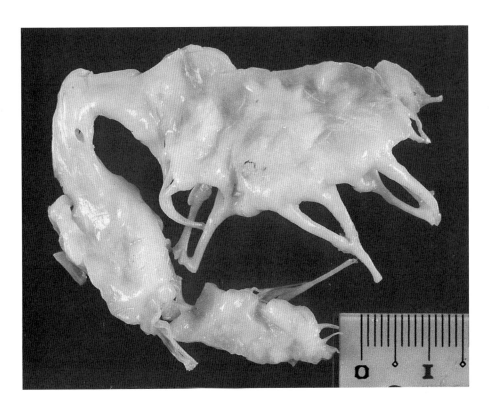

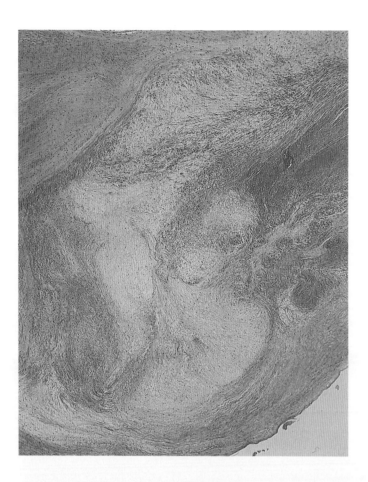

FIG. 72 Mitral valve tissue section from the case discussed in Fig. 71. The upper part shows the atrial surface and the lower part, the ventricular surface. The fibrous layer of the valve leaflet has been replaced by myxomatous tissue. (HE stain, × 10.)

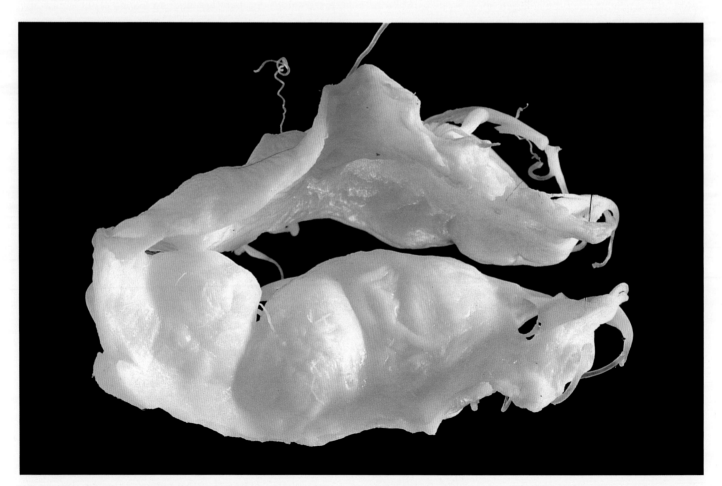

FIG. 73 View from the atrial side of a resected mitral valve of a 32-year-old woman. Heart disease was diagnosed at age 3. At age 15, the patient was diagnosed with Marfan syndrome. At age 29, she developed dyspnea, and cardiomegaly and prolapse of the mitral valve were detected. A dome-shaped protuberance of the posterior leaflet toward the atrium is seen. Fibrotic thickening at the valve margins is present.

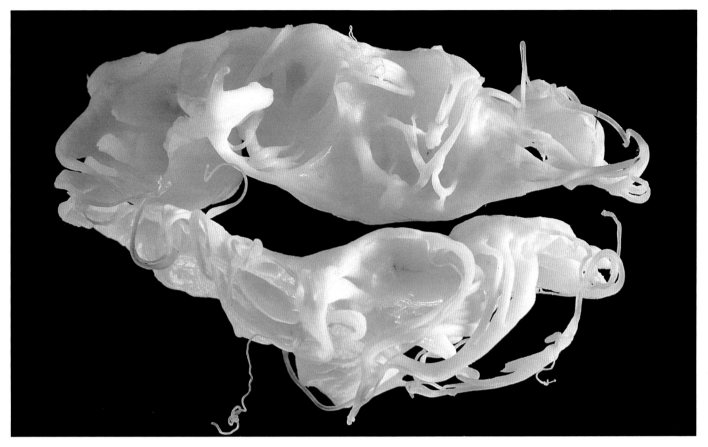

FIG. 74 View from the ventricular side of a resected valve from the case described in Fig. 73 showing abnormal excursion of the chordae tendineae.

FIG. 75 Mitral valve tissue section from the case discussed in Fig. 73. The valve leaflet shows pronounced myxomatous changes, and valve structure is poorly defined. (HE stain, × 10.)

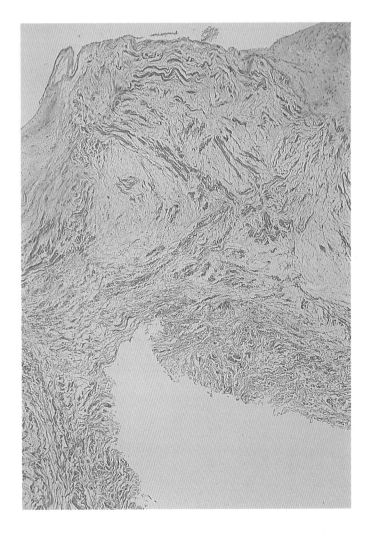

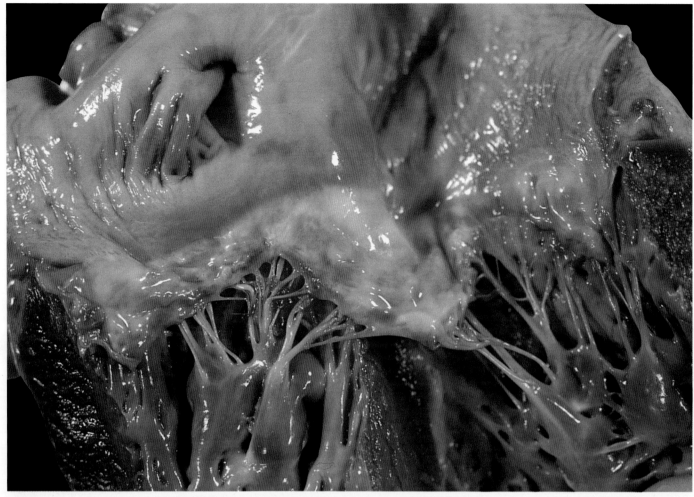

FIG. 76 View of the mitral valve and the left atrium of a 67-year-old man after resection of the posterior wall of the left ventricle (cardiac weight 440 g). At age 48, the patient developed right-sided paresis and dysarthria. At age 58, exertional dyspnea developed, followed at age 65 by the onset of angina-like attacks. Seven days before death, the patient was found in a state of unconsciousness and was admitted on an emergency basis. He subsequently died from cerebral infarction due to thromboembolism. Enlargement of the left atrium and thickening of the wall is shown. On the posterior leaflet of the mitral valve, two scallops protrude in a dome-like shape toward the atrium. The valve leaflets are whitened and opaque, and the supporting chordae tendineae are thin and elongated.

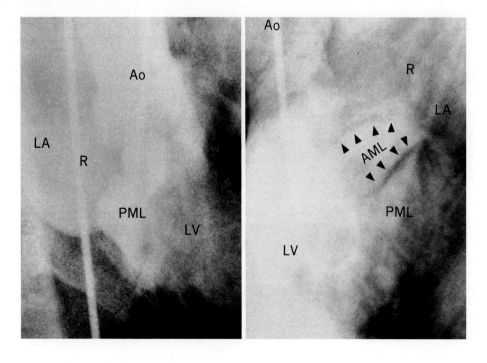

FIG. 77 Angiographic findings. (Left) Left ventriculography (30-degree anterior oblique view). No noticeable prolapse of the posterior leaflet is seen, but there is severe regurgitation. (Right) Marked prolapse of the anterior leaflet toward the atrium (black triangles) (60-degree left anterior oblique view). The posterior leaflet is also prolapsed, and severe regurgitation between the two leaflets is present. (Ao, aorta; LV, left ventricle; PML, posterior mitral leaflet; AML, anterior mitral leaflet; LA, left atrium; R, regurgitation.)

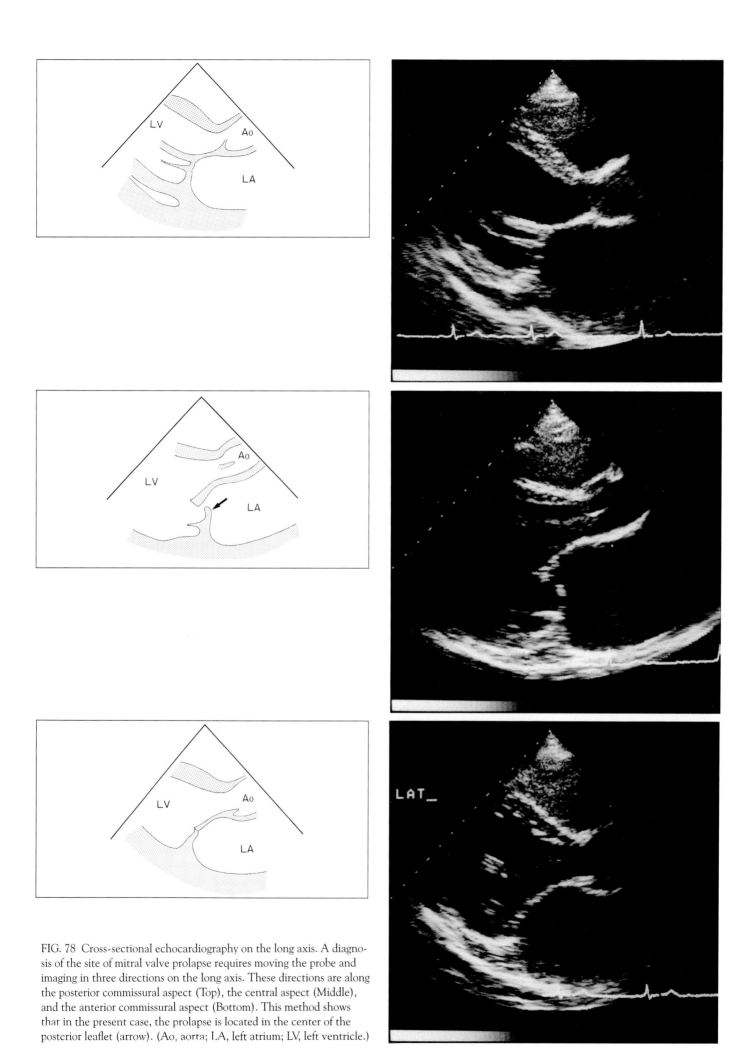

FIG. 78 Cross-sectional echocardiography on the long axis. A diagnosis of the site of mitral valve prolapse requires moving the probe and imaging in three directions on the long axis. These directions are along the posterior commissural aspect (Top), the central aspect (Middle), and the anterior commissural aspect (Bottom). This method shows that in the present case, the prolapse is located in the center of the posterior leaflet (arrow). (Ao, aorta; LA, left atrium; LV, left ventricle.)

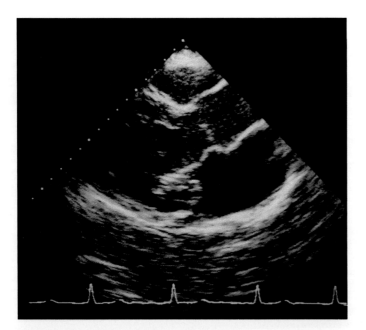

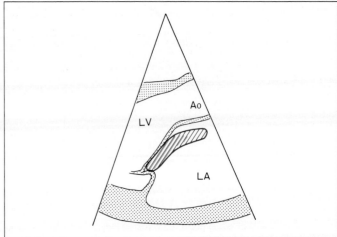

FIG. 79 Cross-sectional echocardiography on the long axis showing displacement of the posterior mitral leaflet toward the left atrium and shearing at the contact surfaces of the anterior and posterior leaflets. The shearing between the anterior and posterior contact surfaces suggests a diagnosis of mitral valve prolapse. (Ao, aorta; LA, left atrium; LV, left ventricle.)

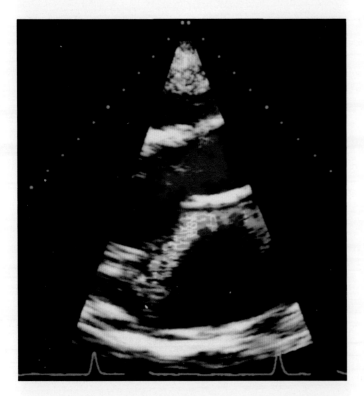

FIG. 80 Two-dimensional Doppler blood flow imaging shows the development of regurgitation from the contact surfaces of the valve in a direction opposite to the damaged valve. (Ao, aorta; LA, left atrium; LV, left ventricle.)

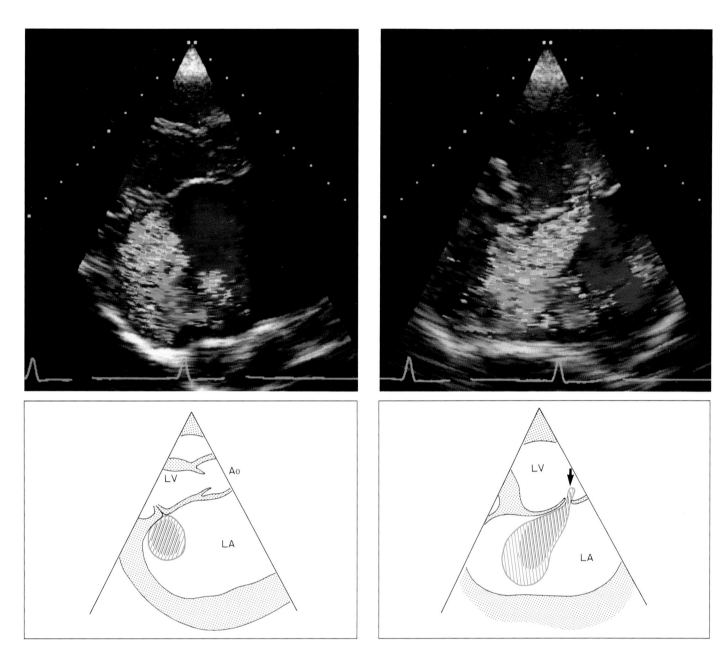

FIG. 81 (Left) Doppler imaging on the long axis of the left ventricle during systole shows a mosaic-like mitral valve regurgitation signal that is recorded in an oval shape from the mitral valve orifice to within the left atrium. This is considered the horizontal cross-section of the regurgitant jet. (Right) The mitral valve cross-section on the short axis records a regurgitant jet originating at the anterior commissural aspect of the mitral valve orifice and moving in a posterior medial direction. Inflow of blood toward the leaky orifice (arrow) is recorded on the left ventricular side of the valve orifice. (Ao, aorta; LA, left atrium; LV, left ventricle.)

FIG. 82 Intraoperative photograph. The mid-section of the valve shows obvious thinning, and there is severe prolapse of the entire anterior leaflet.

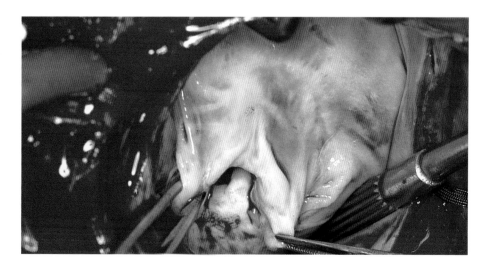

Mitral Valve Prolapse
with Ruptured Chordae

Prolapse frequently occurs at the site of ruptured chordae.

In diagnostic angiography, mitral valve prolapse with ruptured chordae generally shows considerable regurgitation and marked protrusion of the valve into the left atrium. The ruptured chor- dae can be seen flapping between the left ventricle and the left atrium. Echocardiography also shows the ruptured chordae moving freely within the left ventricle during diastole, and can show these ruptured chordae tendineae entering into the left atrium during systole.

For findings using the Doppler method, please refer to the section, "Mitral Valve Prolapse Without Ruptured Chordae."

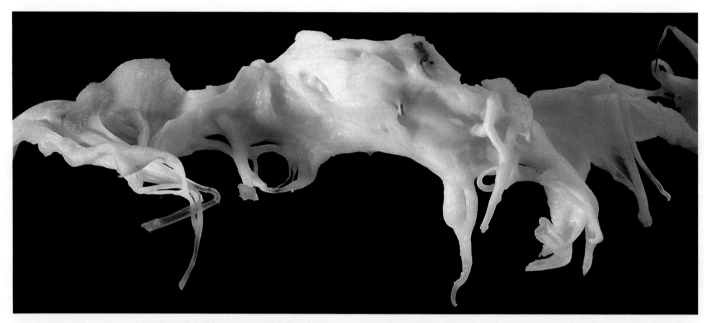

FIG. 83 View from the ventricular side of the posterior leaflet of a resected mitral valve of a 69-year-old man. Heart disease was diagnosed at age 61, orthopnea developed at approximately age 62, and at age 63, a McGoon procedure was performed for mitral valve insufficiency resulting from ruptured chordae. Subsequently, a heart murmur was again detected. Approximately 3 months previously, the patient's heart failure suddenly worsened, and mitral valve replacement and tricuspid valve annuloplasty were performed. Fibrotic thickening of the valve leaflet and fusion and thickening of the chordae tendineae is seen. The blue suture is from previous surgery.

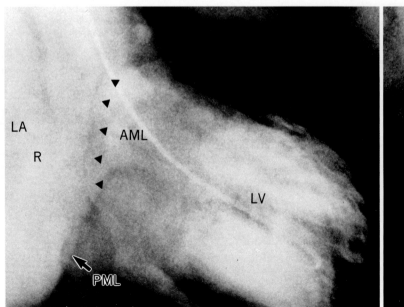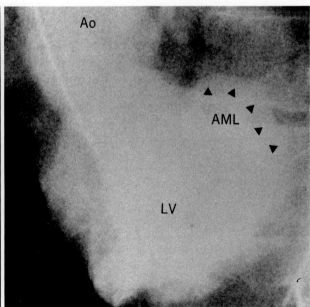

FIG. 84 Angiographic findings. (Left) Left ventriculography (30-degree right anterior oblique) shows extensive prolapse of the anterior leaflet (black triangles) and slight prolapse of the posterior leaflet (black arrow). There is severe regurgitation over an extended area, and the left atrium is markedly enlarged. (Right) The anterior leaflet is markedly distended upward (black triangle … black triangle) due to prolapse (60-degree left anterior oblique view). (AML, anterior mitral leaflet; Ao, aorta; LA, left atrium; LV, left ventricle, PML, posterior mitral leaflet; R, regurgitation.)

Surgical intervention in the form of valvuloplasty involves resection and suturing of the valve leaflet at the ruptured chordae, along with annular plication. This method provides particularly favorable results for ruptured chordae on the posterior leaflet.

Pathologic and morphologic findings are characterized by (1) thickening and transparency in the prolapsed valve and chordae tendineae and (2) in addition to the rupturned chordae, other changes similar to those described in the section "Mitral Valve Prolapse Without Ruptured Chordae."

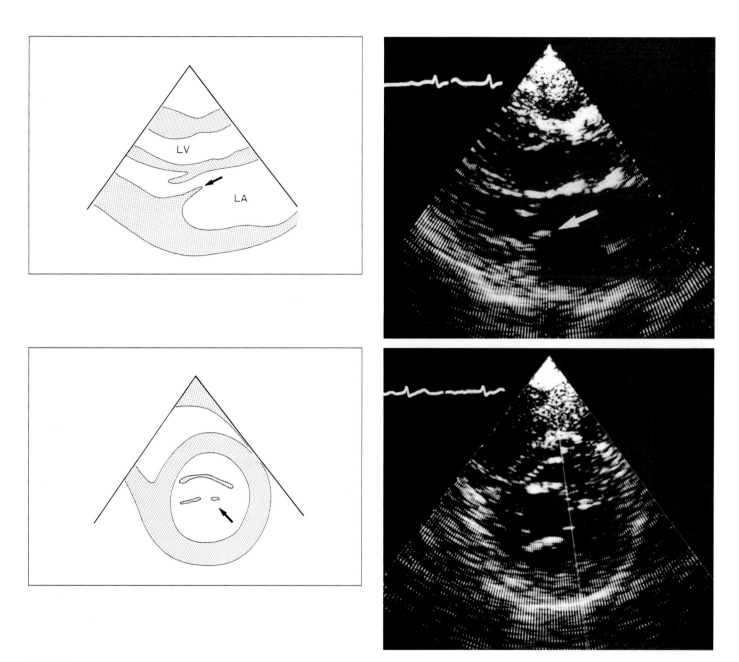

FIG. 85 (Top) Cross-sectional echocardiography on the long axis shows the posterior leaflet of the mitral valve and the fluttering of severed chordae in the left atrium (arrow). (Bottom) Cross-sectional echocardiography on the short axis shows severed chordae on the anterior commissural aspect of the posterior leaflet (arrow). (LA, left atrium; LV, left ventricle.)

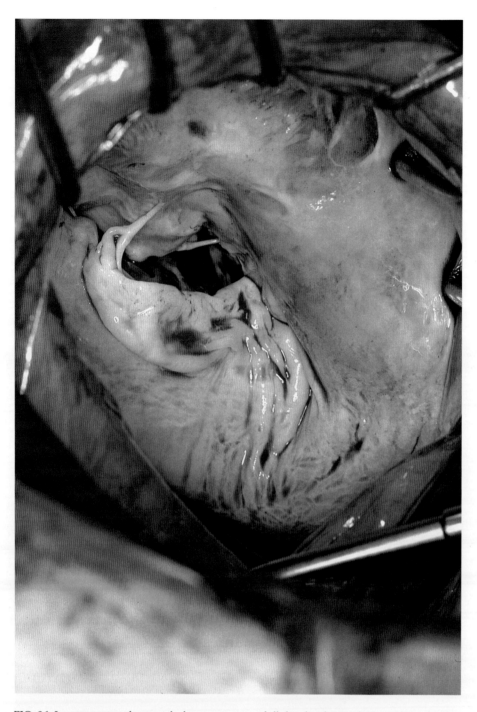

FIG. 86 Intraoperative photograph showing rupture of all the chordae tendineae of the posterior leaflet. There is marked enlargement of the left atrium. The extensive degree of prolapse made valvuloplasty difficult, so a valve replacement procedure was performed.

Mitral Valve Lesion
with Atrial Septal Defect

The primary lesion in this case is prolapse of the posterior commissural aspect of the anterior leaflet.

Diagnostic angiography shows a deep hollow in the upper posterior wall of the left atrium, and characteristic imaging of the left ventricle. Depending on the degree of prolapse, regurgitation may also be present.

Echocardiography of a mitral valve lesion with ostium secundum atrial septal defect shows the posterior commissural aspect of the anterior leaflet; the anterior leaflet deviates toward the left atrium.

For findings from Doppler techniques, please see the section "Mitral Valve Prolapse Without Ruptured Chordae."

Surgical intervention in the form of annular plication and shortening of the chordae in the region of the prolapse has proved highly effective. Valve replacement procedures are not performed for lesions secondary to atrial septal defect.

Pathologic and morphologic findings include (1) fibrosis (induration) of the atrial surface and (2) irregular myxomatous changes.

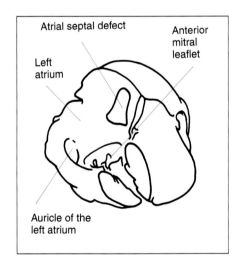

FIG. 87 View of the left atrium and mitral valve of a 62-year-old woman after resection of the posterior walls of the left atrium and left ventricle (cardiac weight 520 g), Heart disease was diagnosed in infancy, but was left untreated. At age 43, the patient developed exertional dyspnea and at age 57, was diagnosed with atrial septal defect. One month before death, her chronic respiratory failure worsened and death ensued. A dome-shaped protuberance of the anterior leaflet of the mitral valve into the left atrium is shown. The protruding portion of the valve leaflet is fibrotic and thickened. Fibrosis is also evidenced in the connected chordae tendineae. The atrium shows a large ostium secundum defect.

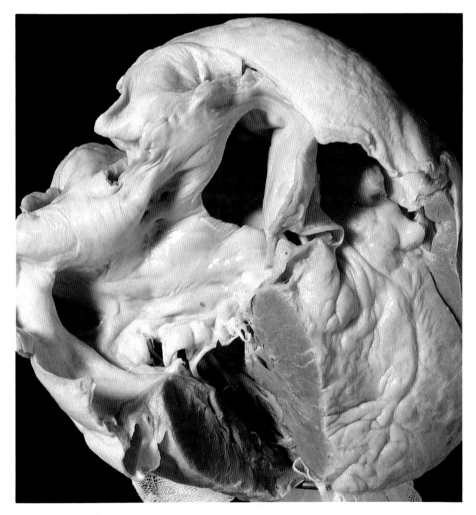

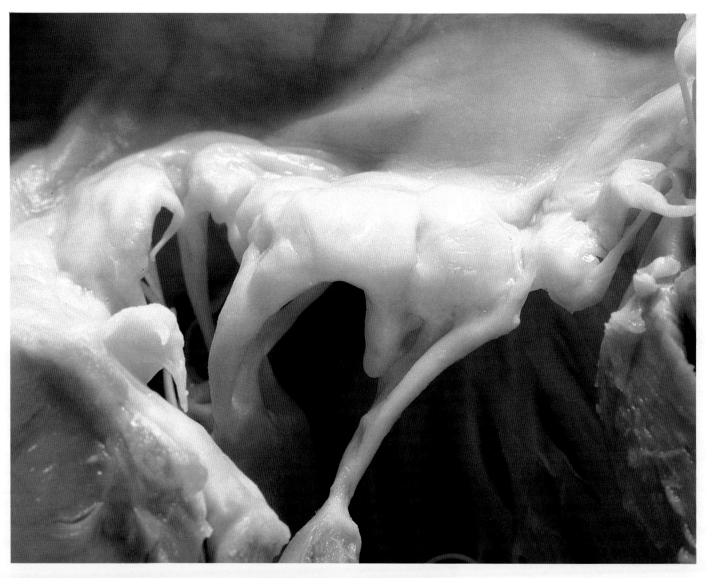

FIG. 88 View of the anterior leaflet of the mitral valve after resection of the posterior wall of the left ventricle of the case discussed in Fig. 87. The valve leaflet protrudes in a dome-like shape toward the atrium; fibrotic thickening is visible at the valve margins. There is pronounced thickening of the chordae tendineae attached to the protruding portion of the valve.

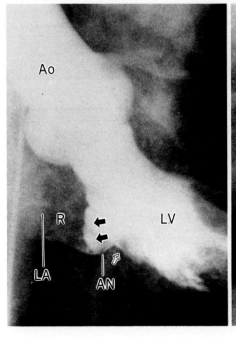
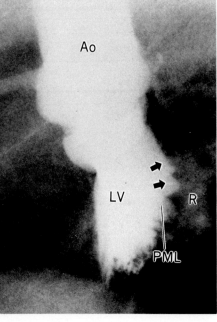

FIG. 89 Angiographic findings. (Left) Left ventriculography (30-degree right anterior oblique view), the anterior leaflet has crossed the valve ring and prolapsed into the left atrium (arrow); mild regurgitation is present. There is visible constriction in the posterior wall of the left ventricle (white arrow). (Right) The anterior leaflet has crossed the posterior leaflet and protrudes posteriorly (arrow); regurgitation is toward the inferior wall of the left atrium (60-degree left anterior oblique view). (AN, annulus; Ao, aorta; LA, left atrium; LV, left ventricle; PML, posterior mitral leaflet; R, regurgitation.)

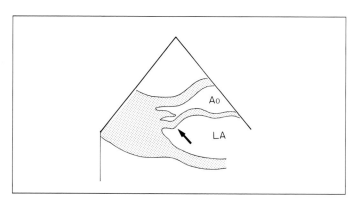

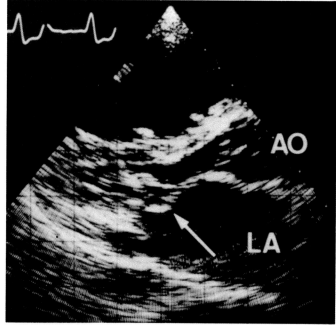

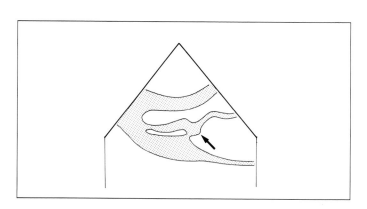

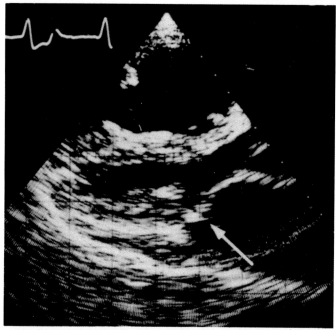

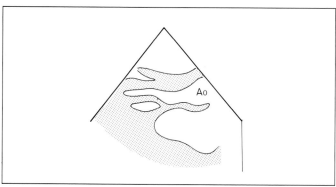

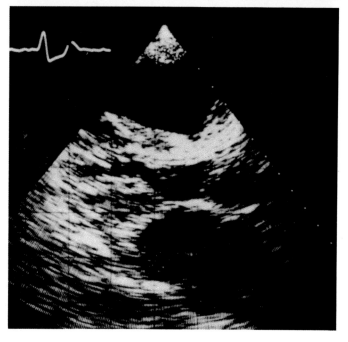

FIG. 90 Cross-sectional echocardiography on the long axis. Imaging is performed in three directions along the long axis. (Top) The posterior commissural aspect of the valve shows shearing at the anterior leaflet. (Middle) The center of the valve also shows abnormalities in the valve. (Bottom) However, the anterior commissural aspect shows no shearing at the anterior leaflet. (Ao, aorta; LA, left atrium.)

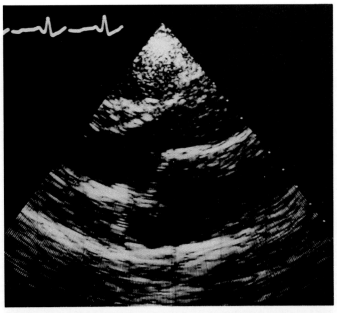
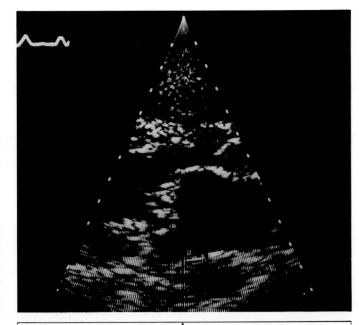
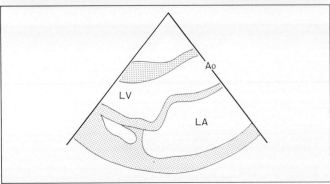

FIG. 91 Cross-sectional echocardiography on the long axis (Left) shows a reversal of the anterior mitral leaflet into the left atrium. (Right) Both the anterior and posterior leaflets enter into the left atrium. Both the anterior and posterior leaflets of the mitral valve are prolapsed. These findings differ from those for mitral valve lesion with ostium secundum atrial septal defect, and should rather be considered indicative of ostium secundum atrial septal defect complicated by idiopathic mitral valve prolapse. (Ao, aorta; LA, left atrium; LV, left ventricle.)

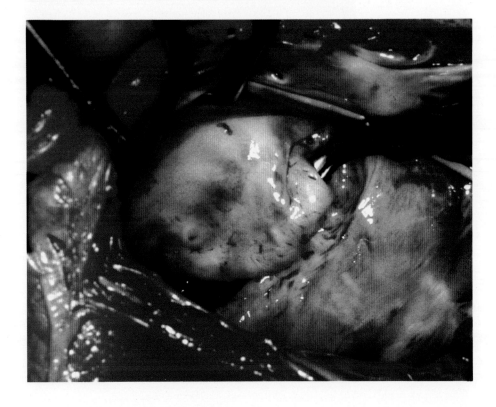

FIG. 92 Intraoperative photograph. Prolapse of the posterior commissure of the anterior leaflet is visible at the point where the forceps are inserted. These are distinctive findings for this condition. Valvuloplasty is performed in similar cases.

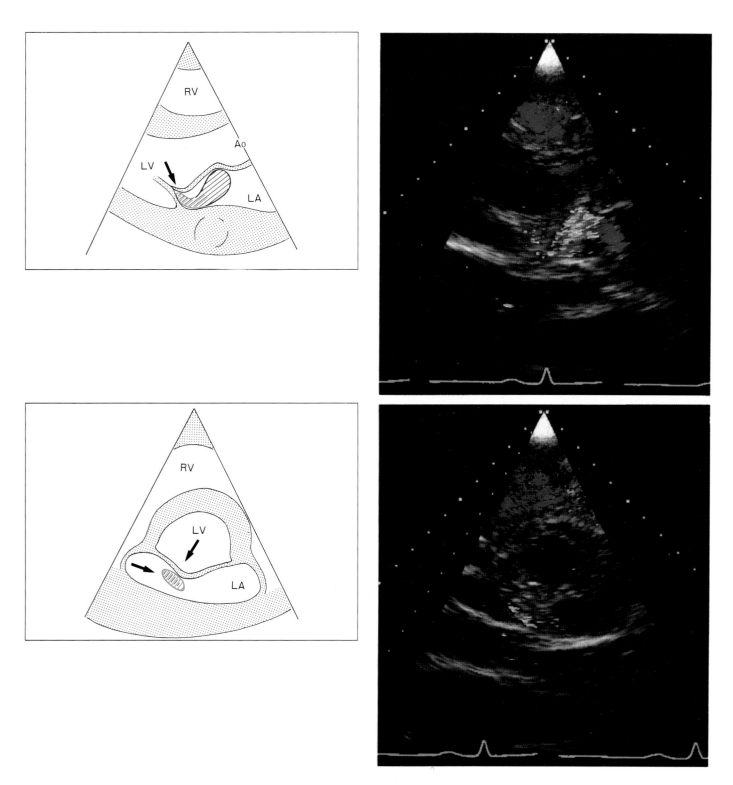

FIG. 93 Doppler imaging. (Top) A somewhat medial cross-sectional view of the left ventricle along the long axis. Mitral valve regurgitation is recorded as a regurgitant jet that travels from the prolapsed portion of the anterior leaflet to the posterior wall of the left atrium, where it is reversed. (Bottom) The cross-section on the short axis of the left ventricle shows prolapse of the anterior leaflet of the mitral valve from the center of the leaflet toward the posterior commissure. The regurgitant signal is recorded from the medial portion of the prolapse. (Ao, aorta; LA, left atrium; LV, left ventricle; RV, right ventricle.)

Infectious Endocarditis

Infectious endocarditis was formerly termed bacterial endocarditis. However, endocarditis can also be caused by fungal infection or by *Rickettsia*, and the condition has recently come to be called *infectious endocarditis*.

Infections may involve both the endocardium and the valve. Infections complicated by patent ductus arteriosus or aortic stenosis are referred to as *arterial endocarditis*. However, with regard to pathogenesis and clinical findings, these infections may be considered under the heading of general infectious endocarditis.

Historically, many cases of subacute endocarditis have been caused by *Streptococcus viridans*, and many cases of acute endocarditis have been caused by *Staphylococcus*. Recently in Japan, *S. viridans* has accounted for the largest number of cases of infectious endocarditis, followed by *Staphylococcus*.

Because *S. viridans* is present within the oral cavity, dental procedures such as tooth extraction and removal of dental calculus provide important pathogenic routes for infection. Other common routes for infection include tonsillectomy, urinary tract procedures, and in recent years heart surgery, cardiac catheterization, and the abuse of intravenous drugs among addicts in Europe and the United States.

A previous history of heart disease can be a factor that causes the patient to be more susceptible to attack by a less virulent bacteria, such as *S. viridans*. Infections by highly pathogenic bacteria, such as *Staphylococcus aureus*, can affect a valve or endocardium that had until then shown no abnormalities. However, in most cases, this infection occurs in subjects with a previous history of valvular heart disease.

Central to the pathophysiology of infectious endocarditis is destruction of the valve mechanism due to inflammation. Vegetations, rupture of the chordae tendineae, or perforation of the valve can exacerbate pre-existing valvular dysfunction. The resulting severe heart failure can be life threatening. It is not uncommon to encounter serious complications, such as emboli from the breaking off of vegetations or intracranial hemorrhage as a result of the rupture of a mycotic aneurysm.

Vegetations

The term *vegetation* indicates a protuberance of essentially anomalous tissue proliferation that is structurally abnormal in appearance. When not accompanying infection, vegetations consist primarily of fibrin, platelets, and small amounts of neutrophils and are smooth on the surface. In the presence of a bacterial or fungal infection, the infiltration of neutrophils increases and there is visible necrosis. The vegetation itself becomes fragile, the surface becomes irregular, and embolization occurs readily. The site of the vegetations varies.

Diagnostic imaging of valvular vegetations is not always straightforward. However, larger vegetations can be observed as negative filling defects at the contact surfaces of the valve.

Echocardiography shows vegetations primarily as abnormal masses on the atrial side of the mitral valve. In some cases they can be seen at the tip of ruptured chordae or on the ventricular side of the anterior leaflet, which is the origin of aortic valve regurgitation.

Surgical intervention in the form of early valve replacement is indicated if the vegetation is clearly in the active stage of formation. However, the presence of a vegetation in the healing stage is rarely sufficient to make the patient a candidate for surgery. In some cases, the same surgical procedures for valvuloplasty are used as described in the section, "Mitral Valve Prolapse with Ruptured Chordae."

Pathologic and morphologic findings are characterized by (1) a stained brittle surface, (2) erosion of valvular tissue, and (3) hemorrhagic necrosis.

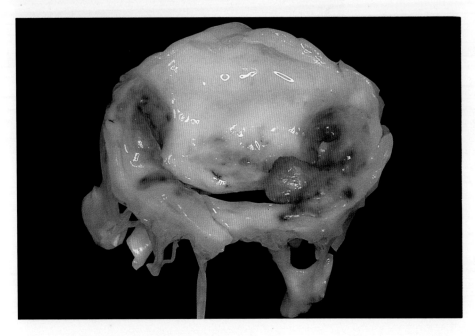

FIG. 94 View from the atrial side of a resected mitral valve of a 37-year-old woman. Four months previously, she developed generalized fatigue. Two and one-half months previously, a fever, heart murmur, and splenomegaly were detected, and spontaneous right hemiplegia developed. Cerebral CT showed subcortical hemorrhaging in the left parietal lobe. Echocardiography revealed vegetations on the mitral valve, and antibiotic treatment was initiated. However, although the patient was maintained on massive doses of antibiotic for a prolonged period, vegetations recurred on the mitral valve and the aortic valve, and mitral and aortic valve replacement procedures were performed. Fibrotic thickening of the valve leaflets and fusion of the commissures indicative of rheumatic valvular disease is shown. The posterior leaflet and the area around the posterior commissure show polyp-shaped protuberances and granular vegetations adhering to the surface. A small vegetation in the region of the anterior commissure is also present.

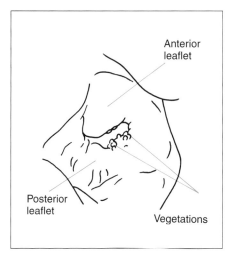

FIG. 95 View of the mitral valve from the atrial cavity (cardiac weight 450 g) of a 72-year-old woman. At age 20, the patient was diagnosed with valvular heart disease. At approximately age 35, she developed exertional dyspnea. Three months before death, dyspnea worsened. α-*Streptococcus* was isolated from blood cultures, and antibiotic treatment was initiated. Because of respiratory complications, the patient was not considered a candidate for surgery. Respiratory failure subsequently worsened and death ensued. A crescent-shaped valve orifice and pronounced fibrotic thickening of the valve leaflets is shown. The anterior leaflet protrudes in a dome shape at the base of the valve. Polyp-shaped formations are visible around the posterior commissure and at the closing margins of the valve, and rough thrombotic vegetations are present on the surface.

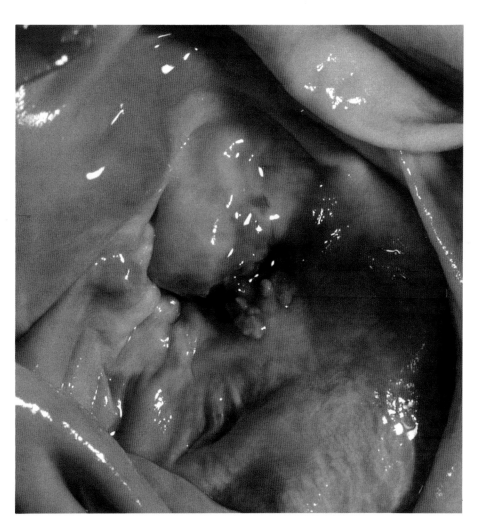

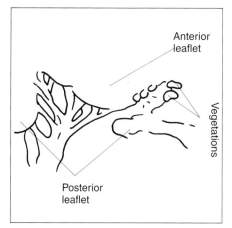

FIG. 96 A view of the mitral valve following dissection of the posterior wall of the left ventricle of the case discussed in Fig. 95. The valve leaflets show fibrotic thickening, and there is fusion of the commissures. The chordae tendineae are fused, shortened, and fibrotic, indicating rheumatic valvular disease. There are thrombotic vegetations on the posterior leaflet and on the closing margins in the region of the posterior commissure. Granular formations are visible on the closing margin of the opposing anterior leaflet.

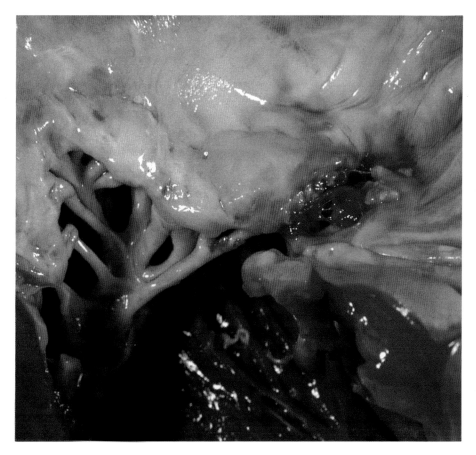

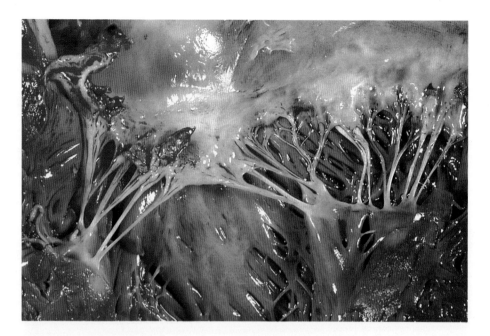

FIG. 97 View of the mitral valve of a 52-year-old man after dissection of the posterior wall of the left ventricle (cardiac weight 575 g). Valvular heart disease was diagnosed at age 47. Three months before death, the patient began to lose weight, and dyspnea developed. Three days before death, echocardiography showed vegetations on the aortic and mitral valves, and antibiotics were given. However, a cerebral hemorrhage developed and death ensued 2 days later. α-Streptococcus was detected in blood cultures. Vegetations with polyp-shaped protrusions adherent to the area around the anterior commissure of the posterior leaflet and the anterior leaflet are shown.

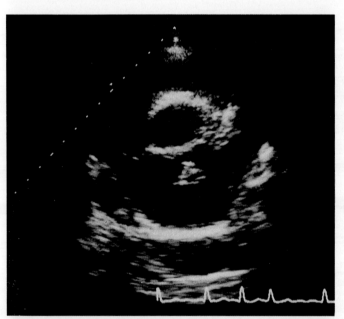

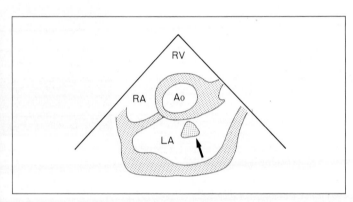

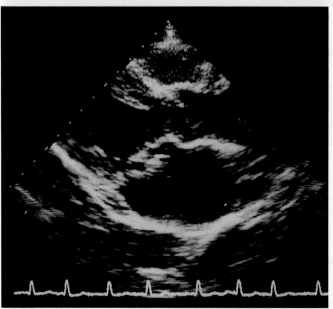

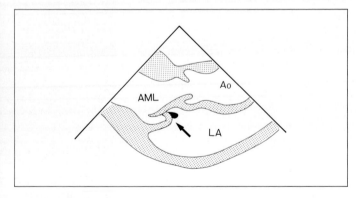

FIG. 98 (Top) Cross-sectional echocardiography on the short axis at the level of the aortic valve shows vegetations within the atrium (arrow). (Bottom) Cross-sectional echocardiography on the long axis shows inversion and prolapse of the posterior mitral leaflet towards the left atrium. Vegetations can be seen on the atrial side of the posterior leaflet (arrow). (Ao, aorta; AML, anterior mitral leaflet; LA, left atrium; RA, right atrium; RV, right ventricle.)

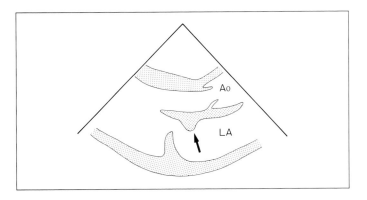
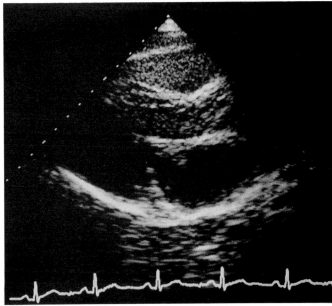

FIG. 99 Cross-sectional echocardiography on the long axis shows vegetations on the anterior mitral leaflet (arrow). (Ao, aorta; LA, left atrium.)

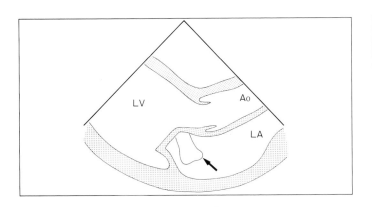
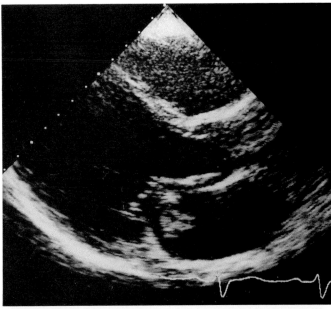

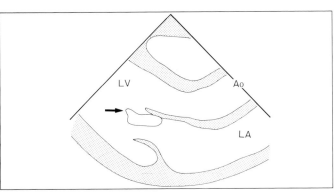
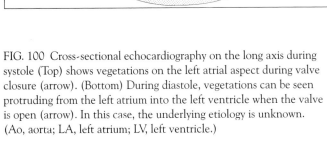
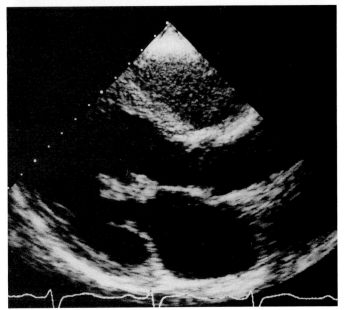

FIG. 100 Cross-sectional echocardiography on the long axis during systole (Top) shows vegetations on the left atrial aspect during valve closure (arrow). (Bottom) During diastole, vegetations can be seen protruding from the left atrium into the left ventricle when the valve is open (arrow). In this case, the underlying etiology is unknown. (Ao, aorta; LA, left atrium; LV, left ventricle.)

Aneurysm and Perforation

In addition to the formation of vegetations, serious complications of infectious endocarditis include aneurysm and perforation. The transition from vegetation to aneurysm formation depends on the pathogenicity of the organism causing the endocarditis. In some cases, the formation of an aneurysm is followed by the development of a perforation. Early diagnosis and treatment (in particular, surgical resection) is desirable in such cases. Valvuloplasty with patching is sometimes an option for the treatment of an aneurysm or perforation during the healing period.

Left ventriculography shows a tumor-like defect protruding into the left atrium during systole. In the presence of a perforation, a regurgitant jet will be visible from the perforation into the atrium.

Echocardiography may show the aneurysm as a partial protrusion of the midsection of the valve into the left atrium. For a perforation, a filling defect in the valve echo is diagnostic.

With the Doppler method, a perforation will be evidenced as a regurgitant jet emitted from the midsection of the valve where it is separated from the original mitral valve orifice during systole. During diastole, a regurgitant jet will be observed from the same location into the left ventricle. It is important in this analysis to differentiate the locations of these abnormal blood flows from the original valve orifice.

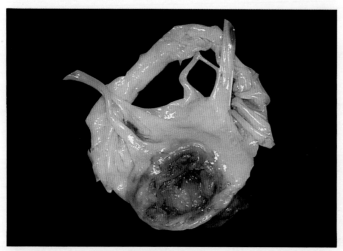
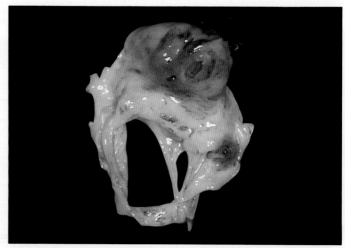

FIG. 101 View of a resected mitral valve from a 29-year-old man. Three weeks previously, the patient developed chills and fever at night and 2 weeks previously, dyspnea, cough, and fever developed. Seven days previously, echocardiography revealed vegetations on the mitral valve. Treatment with antibiotics was initiated, and *Propionibacterium acnes* was detected in blood cultures. The mitral and aortic valves were replaced. A large aneurysm, 2 × 1.5 cm, on the anterior leaflet of the mitral valve and protruding in a dome shape toward the left atrium is seen. The aneurysm is positioned basally from the closing margins of the valve. The ventricular surface of the aneurysm is red-brown with adherent thrombi. The perimeter of the aneurysm is yellow-brown; this color is attributed to mild fibrotic thickening. The remainder of the valve leaflet has retained its transparency, and shows no structural changes. (Left, ventricular side; right, atrial side.)

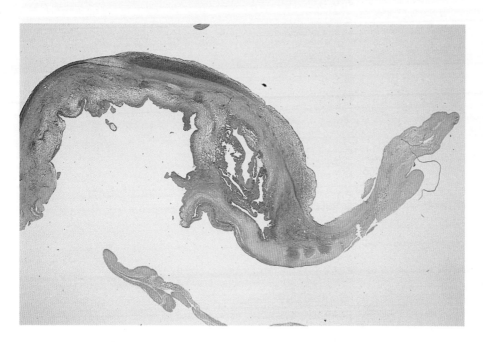

FIG. 102 A tissue section of the mitral valve aneurysm from the case discussed in Fig. 101. The base of the valve protrudes in a dome shape towards the atrium. The atrial surface is relatively smooth, but marked infiltration of inflammatory cells is present. Below, granulation tissue shows visible microvascularization and fibroblastic proliferation. There are thrombi on the ventricular aspect of the section. The upper surface in the figure is the atrial aspect.

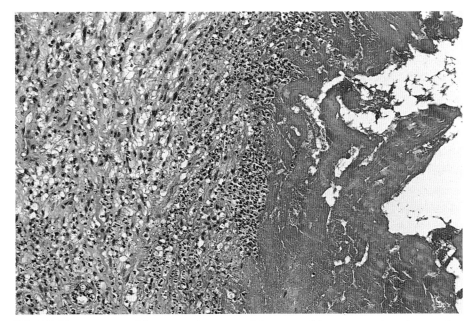

FIG. 103 Tissue section of the ventricular aspect of the origin of the aneurysm from the case discussed in Fig. 101, showing infiltration of inflammatory cells, primarily neutrophils. There is visible proliferation of fibroblasts, and thrombi are present on the ventricular surface. *Propionibacterium acnes* was isolated from blood cultures, but no bacterial colonies were observed in tissue sections from the resected valve. (HE stain, × 175.)

FIG. 104 View of the left atrium and anterior leaflet of the mitral valve of a 34-year-old man after dissection of the posterior wall of the left ventricle (cardiac weight 340 g). Approximately 1 month previously, the patient developed a fever. Three weeks previously, he was diagnosed by his personal physician with pneumonia and endocarditis, and treatment was initiated. However, 16 days previously, his respiratory condition worsened. *Staphylococcus aureus* and *Streptococcus faecalis* were isolated from blood cultures. Echocardiography showed vegetations on the mitral valve, and intensive antibiotic therapy was initiated, but the patient developed adult respiratory distress syndrome (ARDS) and died. An aneurysm on the anterior mitral leaflet, approximately 2 cm in diameter, that extends from the valve margin to the base of the valve and protrudes in a dome shape toward the atrial side is shown. The aneurysm is yellow-brown. The surface is granular, and thrombi are present. A perforation is visible near the valve margin.

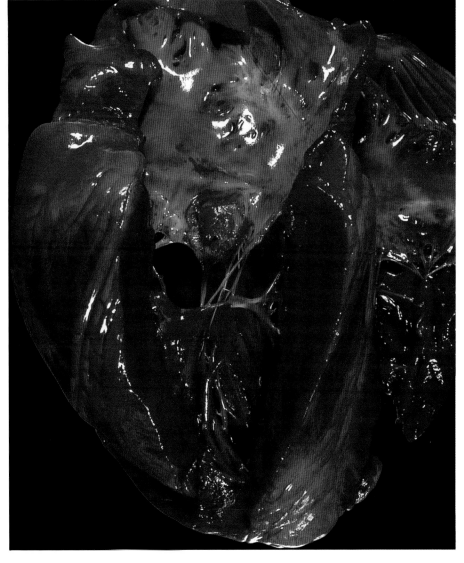

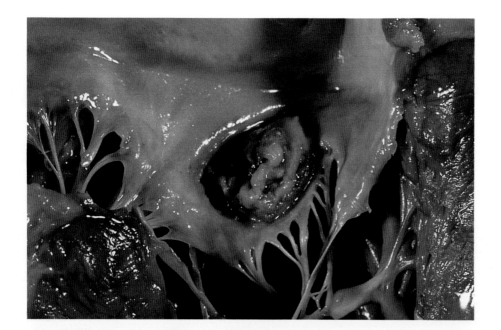

FIG. 105 View of the mitral valve from the case discussed in Fig. 104, after preservation in formalin. The aneurysm protruding into the atrial side is more indented than at the time of autopsy. The surface is granular, with a yellow tone, and thrombi are present. The aneurysm extends from the valve margin to the base of the valve. The other areas of the valve leaflet have retained their transparency. No predisposing structural damage is evident. A perforation is visible near the valve margin.

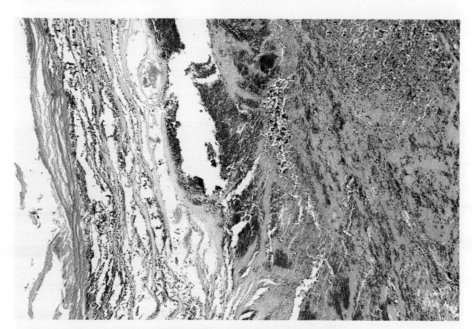

FIG. 106 Tissue section of the aneurysm from the case discussed in Fig. 104. The left side shows the atrial surface of the aneurysm. Numerous bacteria are visible as blue-violet stained aggregations. *Escherichia coli, Enterobacter aerogenes, Streptococcus faecalis, α-Streptococcus,* and *Bacteroides* sp. were isolated from cultures done at autopsy. Adherent thrombi are visible on the right. Although numerous bacteria are visible, there is only very mild infiltration by inflammatory cells. (HE stain, × 175.)

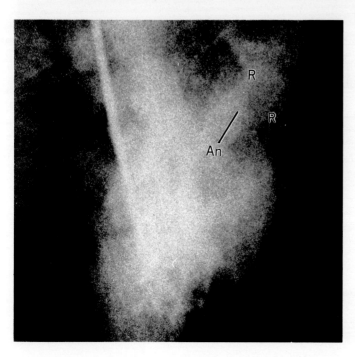

FIG. 107 Angiographic findings show pronounced aneurysm formation in the mitral valve and severe regurgitation. (An, aneurysm; R, regurgitation.)

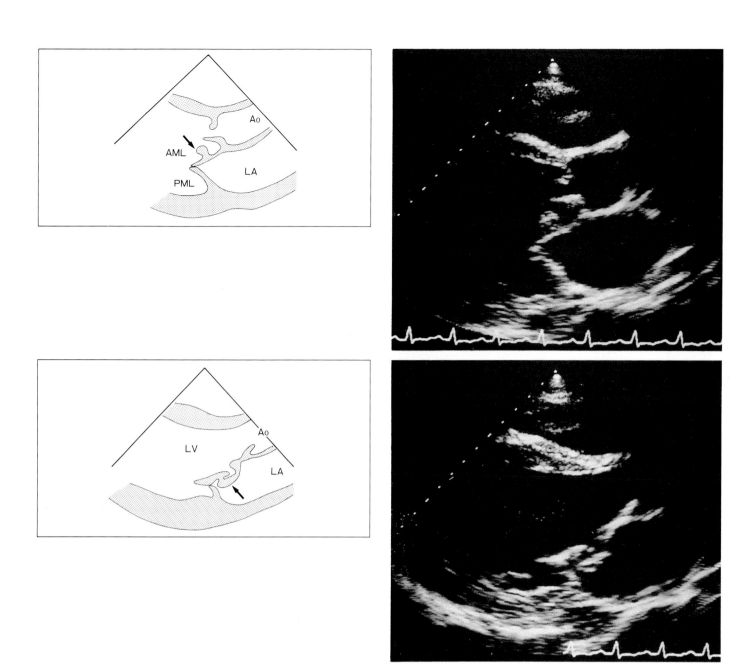

FIG. 108 (Top) Cross-sectional echocardiography on the long axis during diastole shows a mitral aneurysm on the left ventricular side (arrow). The aortic valve has fallen into the left ventricle. (Bottom) Cross-sectional echocardiography on the long axis during systole shows that the mitral valve annulus has shifted toward the left atrium (arrow). These findings do not provide sufficient information to determine whether the aneurysm has perforated. The aortic valve, visible on the ventricular side during diastole, is seen on the aortic side during systole. (AML, anterior mitral leaflet; Ao, aorta; LA, left atrium; LV, left ventricle; PML, posterior mitral leaflet.)

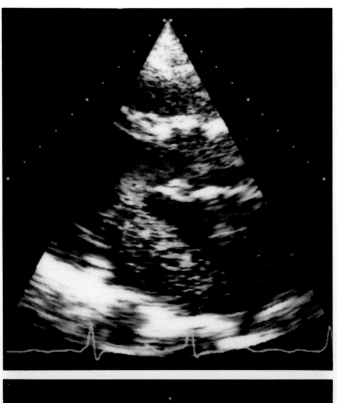
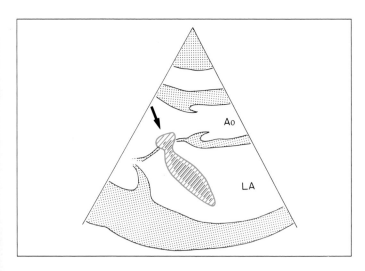
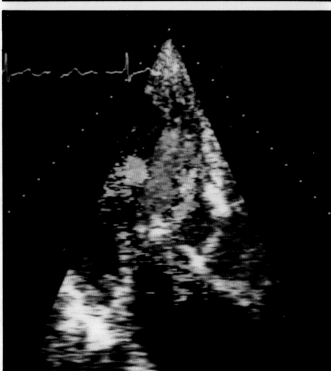
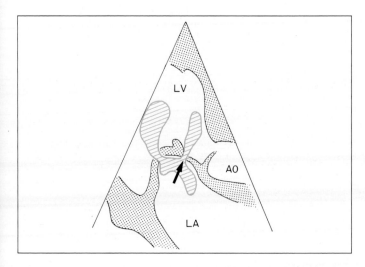

FIG. 109 Doppler imaging. (Top) Parasternal left ventricular cross-section on the long axis during systole. A blue and mosaic-patterned abnormal blood flow signal is recorded passing through the mitral valve from the left atrial aspect and the left ventricular aspect of the central midsection (arrow) of the anterior mitral leaflet. This is attributed to regurgitation through the anterior mitral leaflet. (Bottom) Apical left ventricular cross-section on the long axis during diastole. Left ventricular inflow during diastole is recorded as a red-yellow signal that shows two abnormal inflows from the mitral valve orifice (left side of figure) and the central midsection of the anterior mitral leaflet (arrow). The signal indicated by the arrow in the diagram is attributed to blood flow through a perforation in the anterior leaflet. (Ao, aorta; LA, left atrium; LV, left ventricle.)

Mitral Regurgitation Caused by Myocardial Disease

Even if no structural changes of the mitral valve itself are present, mitral regurgitation can develop from a number of etiologies, including diseases of the myocardium. In particular, dilated and hypertrophic cardiomyopathies are discussed.

Dilated cardiomyopathy is characterized by marked dilation of the left ventricle and thinning of the ventricular wall. These factors often result in dilation of the mitral valve annulus and/or abnormalities of the supporting tissues of the mitral valve, leading to regurgitation.

In mitral regurgitation associated with dilated cardiomyopathy, diagnostic imaging often reveals a wide rather than jet-like regurgitant flow.

Echocardiography shows gaps and shearing at the contact surfaces of the valve as a result of enlargement of the mitral valve annulus and papillary muscle dysfunction, with subsequent development of mitral regurgitation.

Because hypertrophic cardiomyopathy is associated with myocardial hypertrophy and marked narrowing of the left ventricular cavity, regurgitation is thought to occur as a result of systolic anterior motion of the mitral valve. Subaortic fibrotic thickening is present in this condition.

In hypertrophic cardiomyopathy, diagnostic imaging shows trapping of contrast medium in the cardiac apex by the papillary muscles. Imaging may also show a spade-like configuration of the left ventricle at the end of systole.

Echocardiography shows regurgitation resulting from deformation of the mitral valve due to systolic anterior motion of the valve.

For the treatment of mitral regurgitation associated with dilated cardiomyopathy, valvuloplasty (annular plication) is sometimes performed. In hypertrophic cardiomyopathy, surgical intervention is not only indicated for mitral regurgitation, but also to relieve left ventricular outflow obstruction. Surgical intervention corrects the anterior motion of the mitral valve through dissection and resection of the hypertrophied septal myocardium. This procedure also relieves outflow obstruction and eliminates mitral regurgitation.

The above findings can involve the anterior leaflet, the posterior leaflet, or both leaflets of the mitral valve. The following pathologic and morphologic findings are characteristic: (1) fibrosis of the atrial surfaces, (2) irregular myxomatous degeneration, (3) abnormal motion of the papillary muscles, (4) dilation of the mitral valve annulus (in dilated cardiomyopathy), and (5) subaortic endocardial fibrosis (in obstructive hypertrophic cardiomyopathy).

FIG. 110 View after dissection of the posterior wall of the left ventricle (cardiac weight 690 g) of a 37-year-old man. At age 28, cardiomegaly was detected, and at age 32, dilated cardiomyopathy was diagnosed. Although the patient received treatment, he gradually developed worsening heart failure over the next 5 years and subsequently died. Marked dilation of the left ventricular cavity is shown. A portion of the endocardium appears white and shows fibrotic thickening. The mitral valve annulus is enlarged, and the valve leaflets have thinned. Part of the posterior leaflet demonstrates dome-like protrusion into the left atrium.

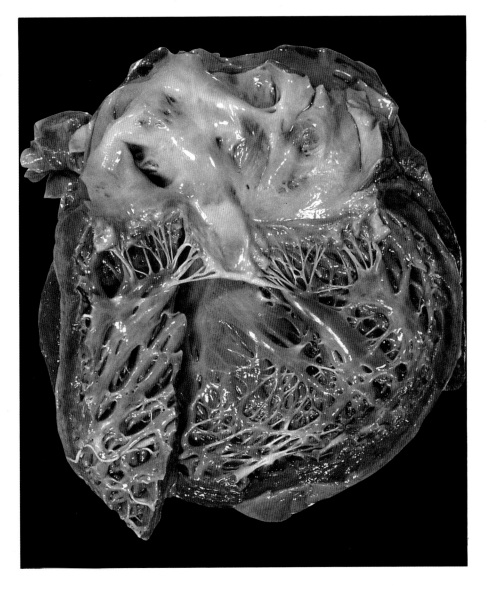

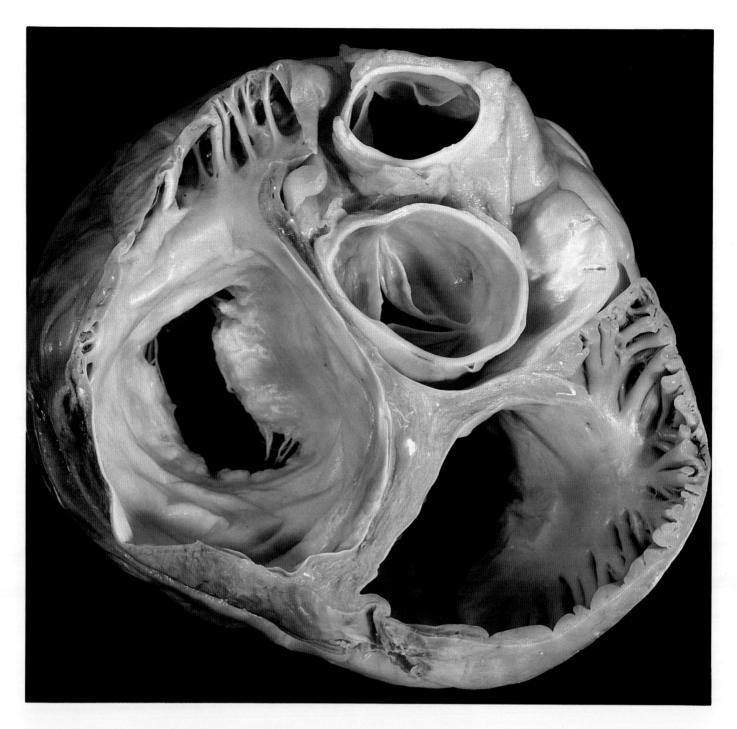

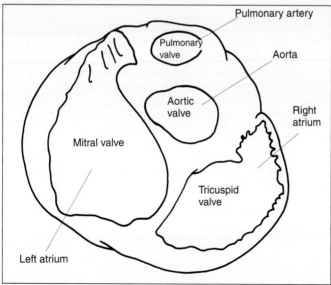

FIG. 111 View of the four valves after resection of the right and left atria (cardiac weight 550 g) of a 57-year-old man. At age 47, cardiomegaly was detected, and at age 53, atrial fibrillation was diagnosed. Two weeks before death, he developed generalized fatigue. An abnormality was detected on electrocardiogram by his primary physician. Eleven days before death, the patient developed a cerebral infarction, and subsequently died. Dilation of the mitral valve annulus is seen. The left atrium is also dilated.

FIG. 112 View of the mitral valve from the atrial side of the case discussed in Fig. 111. The anterior leaflet is seen at the top. Although the valve margins show mild fibrotic thickening, the remainder of the valve maintains its translucency. The chordae tendineae show no notable changes.

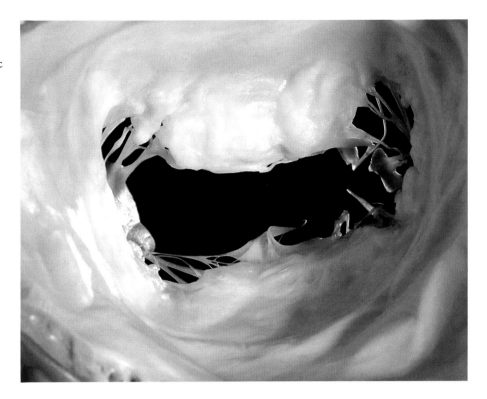

FIG. 113 Anterior view of the left ventricular outflow tract (cardiac weight 770 g; interventricular septum/posterior wall ratio, 1.5:1.0) of a 36-year-old man. At age 17, an arrhythmia was detected. At age 28, the patient experienced the onset of exertional dyspnea, and at age 30, a heart murmur was audible. Hypertrophic cardiomyopathy was diagnosed at age 31. One year before death, the patient developed symptoms of heart failure. His condition gradually deteriorated and death ensued. Narrowing of the left ventricular cavity and subaortic fibrotic thickening is seen.

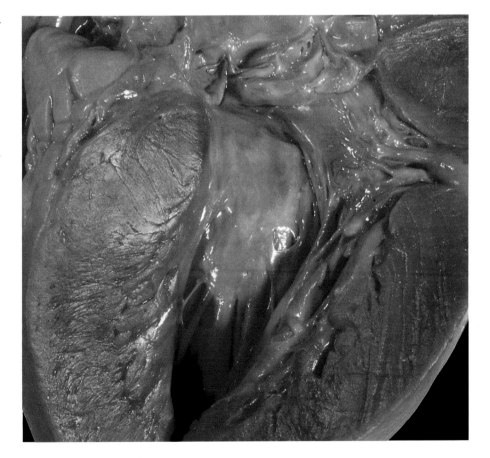

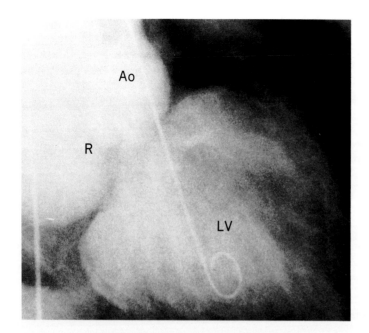

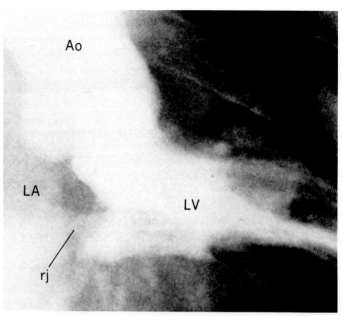

FIG. 114 Angiographic findings (dilated cardiomyopathy). Left ven-triculography (30-degree right anterior oblique) demonstrates an enlarged left ventricle and the development of severe mitral regurgitation from the mitral valve annulus. (Ao, aorta; LV, left ventricle; R, regurgitation.)

FIG. 115 Angiographic findings (hypertrophic cardiomyopathy). Left ventriculography (30-degree right anterior oblique) shows the development of a regurgitant jet from the posterior medial commissure of the mitral valve. There is a moderate degree of regurgitation. (Ao, aorta; LA, left atrium; LV, left ventricle; rj, regurgitant jet.)

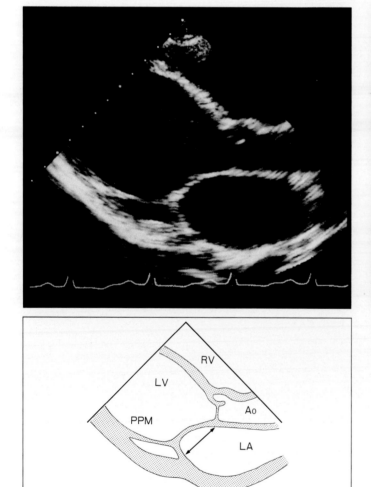

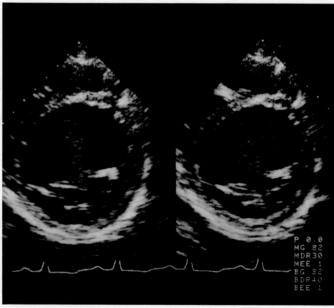

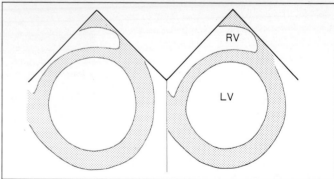

FIG. 116 Echocardiography (dilated cardiomyopathy). (Left) Cross-sectional echocardiography on the long axis shows dilation of the mitral valve annulus (arrow) with associated papillary muscle dysfunction. No abnormalities are visible in the contact areas of the mitral valve. (Right)

Cross-sectional echocardiography along the short axis (left panel, during diastole; right panel, during systole) reveals left ventricular dilation and incomplete cardiac contractility. (Ao, aorta; LA, left atrium; LV, left ventricle; PPM, posterior papillary muscle; RV, right ventricle.)

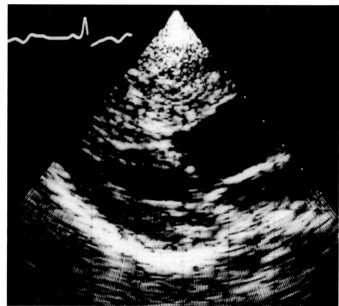

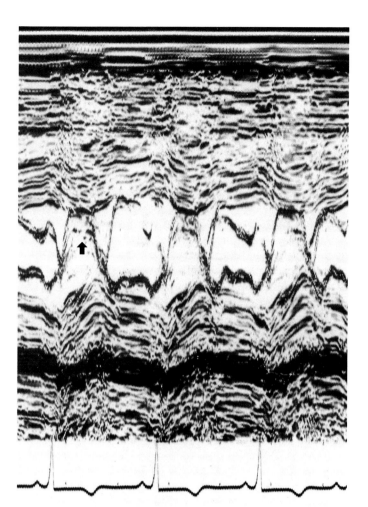

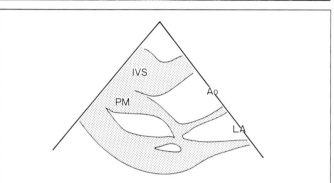

FIG. 117 Echocardiography (hypertrophic obstructive cardiomyopathy). (Left) Cross-sectional echocardiography along the long axis shows deviation of the hypertrophied papillary muscle toward the interventricular septum, causing the chordae tendineae and the mitral valve to also shift toward the interventricular septum. This deformity of the mitral valve leads to mitral insufficiency. (Right) M-mode echocardiography demonstrates systolic anterior motion of the mitral valve (arrow). (Ao, aorta; IVS, interventricular septum; LA, left atrium; PM, papillary muscle.)

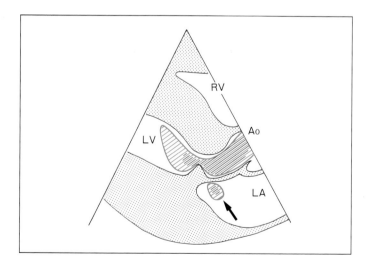

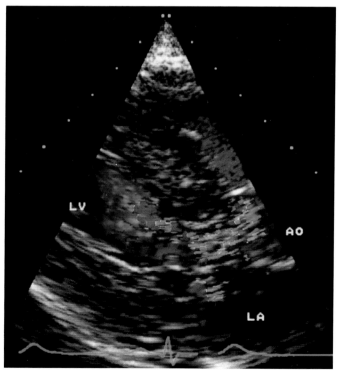

FIG. 118 Doppler imaging. A cross-section on the long axis of the left ventricle during systole shows prominent thickening of the left ventricular wall. There is constriction of the left ventricular cavity at the level from the mitral valve leaflets to the chordae tendineae. A mosaic-like pattern of abnormal blood flow is demonstrated from this area to the outflow tract. There is a mild degree of mitral regurgitation (arrow) from the portion of the mitral valve orifice in contact with this area into the left atrium. (Ao, aorta; LA, left atrium; LV, left ventricle; RV, right ventricle.)

Papillary Muscle Dysfunction

Papillary muscle dysfunction was first discussed by Burch and colleagues in 1963. In this condition, abnormal contraction or rupture of the papillary muscles, with associated mitral regurgitation, may result from various etiologies.

The most common cause of this disorder is ischemic cardiovascular insufficiency. Papillary muscle dysfunction may be transient, with mitral insufficiency occurring only during episodes of angina pectoris. Myocardial infarction, however, may result in new and old infarct-related lesions of the papillary muscles, such as myocardial necrosis, fibrosis, and calcification. In most instances there is some degree of persistent mitral insufficiency. In the narrow meaning of papillary muscle dysfunction as seen in the broader context of ischemic heart disease or dilated cardiomyopathy, this dysfunction is caused by a lack of contractile coordination between the left ventricular wall and the papillary muscles. Such lack of coordination can result from separation of the relative position bilaterally of the papillary muscles that accompanies dilation of the left ventricular cavity, leading to further abnormal separation during systole, but may also be due to conduction disturbances or premature ventricular contractions.

Papillary muscle necrosis is reported to occur in 10% to 50% of cases of acute myocardial infarction. Acute regurgitation is said to develop in 15% of cases of anterior wall infarction, and in 40% of cases of posterior wall infarction. Regurgitation due to papillary muscle rupture is very rare.

Papillary muscle dysfunction should be suspected when, despite a limited area of involvement of myocardial infarction, there is severe valvular insufficiency but a relatively normal ejection fraction on left ventriculography, or in cases in which, despite the absence of a ventricular aneurysm, there is low cardiac output. If a regurgitant jet is demonstrated in these circumstances, a diagnosis of papillary muscle dysfunction is likely.

Echocardiographic findings of changes in the papillary muscles (primarily fibrosis) or detection of left ventricular wall motion abnormalities at the site of attachment of the papillary muscles are important in diagnosis.

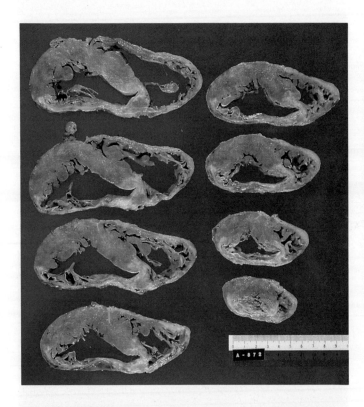

FIG. 119 View of the left and right ventricles with coronal sections at 1-cm intervals, starting from the apex (cardiac weight 505 g), of a 73-year-old man. At age 68, the patient suffered an inferior wall myocardial infarction complicated by mitral regurgitation. At age 71, rupture of the chordae tendineae resulted in exacerbation of mitral regurgitation. Heart failure subsequently continued to worsen and death ensued. Thinning of the posterior septum and posterior wall of the left ventricle as a result of myocardial infarction is shown. Normal tissue has been replaced with fibrous tissue. The posterior medial papillary muscle group demonstrates fibrosis and atrophy.

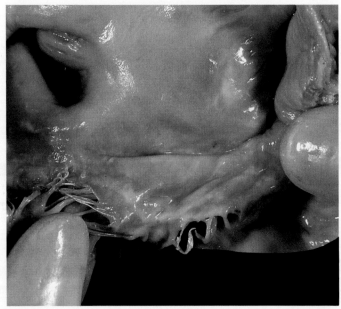

FIG. 120 View of the mitral valve after dissection of the posterior wall of the left ventricle from the case discussed in Fig. 119. There is visible folding of the posterior aspect of the mitral valve anterior leaflet. The chordae tendineae attached to the posterior medial papillary muscle group are ruptured.

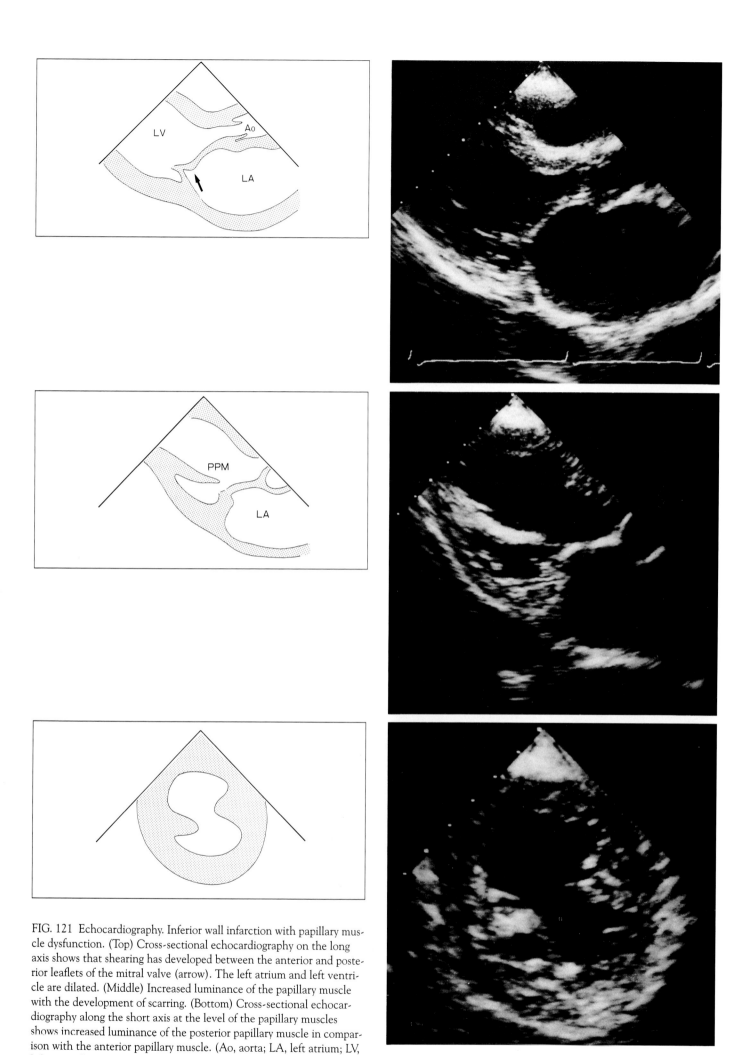

FIG. 121 Echocardiography. Inferior wall infarction with papillary muscle dysfunction. (Top) Cross-sectional echocardiography on the long axis shows that shearing has developed between the anterior and posterior leaflets of the mitral valve (arrow). The left atrium and left ventricle are dilated. (Middle) Increased luminance of the papillary muscle with the development of scarring. (Bottom) Cross-sectional echocardiography along the short axis at the level of the papillary muscles shows increased luminance of the posterior papillary muscle in comparison with the anterior papillary muscle. (Ao, aorta; LA, left atrium; LV, left ventricle; PPM, posterior papillary muscle.)

Mitral Valve Cleft

Mitral valve cleft is a rare anomaly of the mitral valve leaflets. This condition is seen with congenital endocardial cushion defects. It is not associated with defects involving a common atrioventricular orifice. The cleft usually involves the anterior leaflet and can result in valvular insufficiency. Although surgical repair of the cleft is often sufficient, shortening of the chordae tendineae or plication of the valve annulus (or both) is sometimes necessary.

Left ventriculography (frontal view) shows the mitral valve located to the left of its normal position. The left ventricular outflow tract is elongated. Although there is no common atrioven-tricular orifice, there is a gooseneck deformity. The anterior leaflet of the mitral valve has a serrated appearance (scalloping) during systole. There is a band-like filling defect resulting from the cleft in the central portion of the leaflet. It is from this area that the regurgitant jet arises.

Cross-sectional echocardiography along the short axis shows findings consistent with the anterior leaflet dividing into right and left sections with opening of the mitral valve. Doppler studies show a regurgitant jet along the cleft of the mitral valve anterior leaflet. Abnormal blood flow is recorded along the left ventricular side of the cleft during systole.

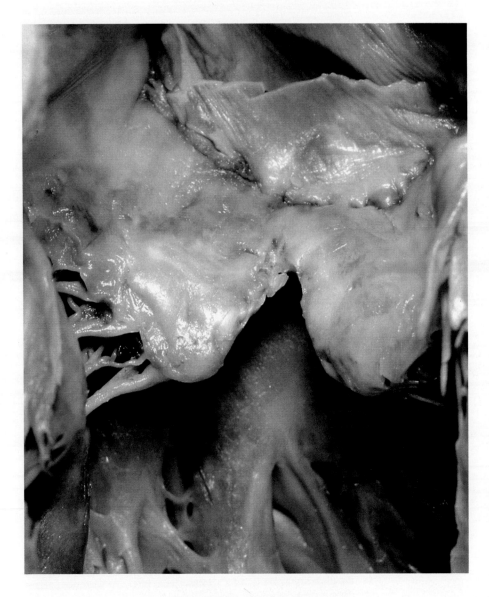

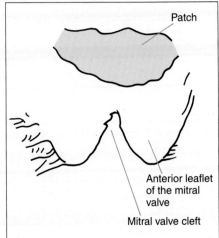

FIG. 122 View of the anterior leaflet of the mitral valve of a 41-year-old woman after dissection of the left ventricle. At approximately age 33, she had the onset of occasional syncopal attacks. Two months previously, cardiomegaly and an arrhythmia were detected by her personal physician. An endocardial cushion defect with complete atrioventricular block was diagnosed. A large cleft in the central part of the anterior leaflet is shown. Above this was a large foramen primum atrial septal defect, which was closed with a patch.

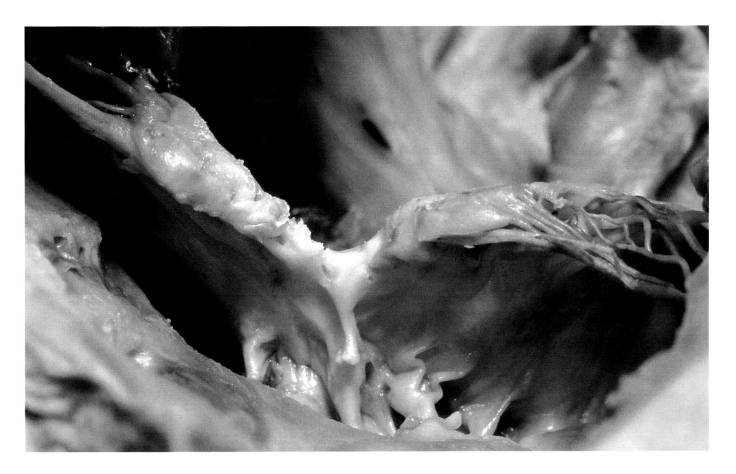

FIG. 123 View from the ventricular side of the mitral valve cleft of the case discussed in Fig. 122. The chordae tendineae show mild thickening.

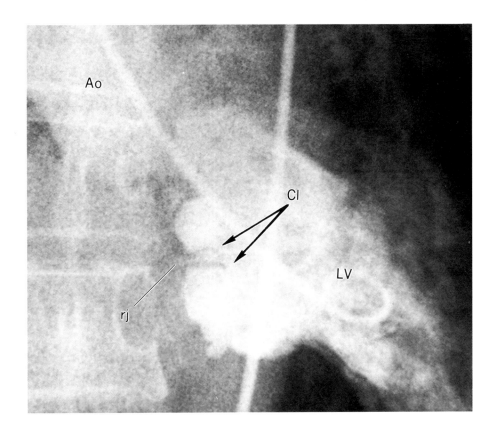

FIG. 124 Left ventriculography (frontal view) shows an incomplete endocardial cushion defect and a regurgitant jet from the cleft of the thickened anterior leaflet of the mitral valve into the left atrium. (Ao, aorta; Cl, cleft; LV, left ventricle; rj, regurgitant jet.)

Mitral Valvular Disease 87

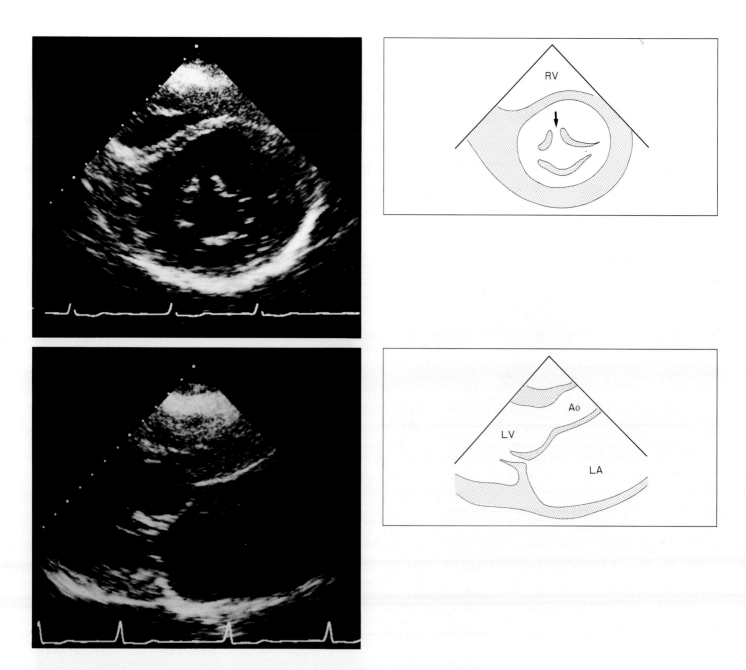

FIG. 125 (Top) Cross-sectional echocardiography along the short axis shows a cleft in the central portion of the mitral valve anterior leaflet (arrow). (Bottom) Cross-sectional echocardiography on the long axis shows shearing between the anterior and posterior leaflets of the mitral valve. There is also annular dilation. (Ao, aorta; LA, left atrium; LV, left ventricle; RV, right ventricle.)

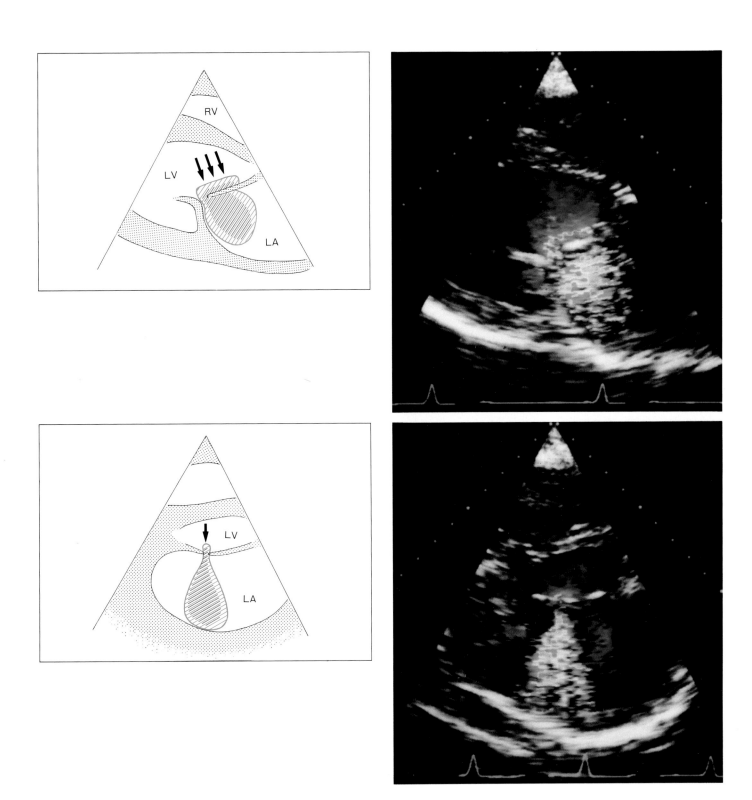

FIG. 126 Doppler imaging. (Top) A cross-section on the long axis of the left ventricle during systole records a wide regurgitant jet from the anterior leaflet of the mitral valve into the left atrium. There is a wide abnormal signal along the left ventricular side of the mitral valve anterior leaflet. (Bottom) A cross-section along the short axis of the left ventricle shows rupture in the center of the mitral valve. A wide regurgitant jet originating from this area is recorded. The location and width of the cleft can be estimated based on this rectangular regurgitant jet seen from the left ventricle into the left atrium. (LA, left atrium; LV, left ventricle; RV, right ventricle.)

Mitral Annular Calcification

It is estimated that mitral annular calcification is found in about 10% of autopsy cases in which the patient was age 50 or older. Mitral annular calcification is three times more common in women than in men, and its prevalence increases with age.

The initial lesions develop in the central or commissural regions of the posterior leaflet. If the length of the calcification is 30 mm or longer, valvular insufficiency will develop. The probable mechanism is that calcifications arising on the posterior leaflet, at its attachment to the heart, elevate the valve and restrict the range of valvular excursion.

Mitral annular calcification is often associated with diabetes, osteitis deformans, and metastatic calcification. This condition is also thought to occur in the absence of other underlying disorders or in association with age-related degenerative diseases.

Chest radiographs can show mitral annular calcification. In cases in which there is severe calcification covering the entire valve annulus, the presence of ring-like calcified shadows is diagnostic. However, the thick and overlapping shadows of the heart often present difficulties in radiographic interpretation. Small calcifications are readily visible under fluoroscopy or cineangiography.

Echocardiography is the most useful method of diagnosing this condition. It detects ring-like echoes with enhanced luminance of the valve ring at the site of attachment of the posterior leaflet.

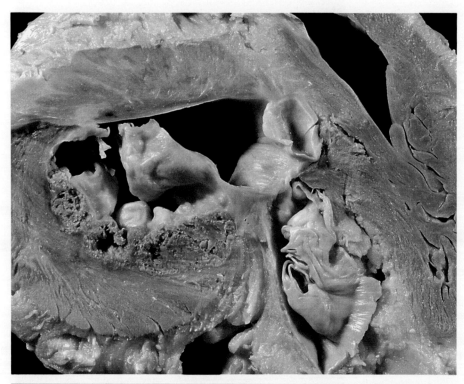

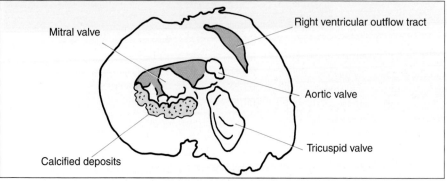

FIG. 127 Horizontal cross-sectional view of the mitral valve annulus (cardiac weight 515 g) of a 74-year-old woman. At age 56, she was diagnosed with hypertension and myxedema by her personal physician and treatment was initiated. Fifteen days before death, the patient suffered an acute myocardial infarction. Heart failure developed and the patient subsequently died. Aggregated calcified deposits just beneath the mitral valve and extending partially into the myocardium are shown. These calcified deposits extend halfway around the valve ring in a J-shaped configuration. There are no marked changes in the mitral valve itself. An extensive area of myocardial infarction, primarily subendocardial, is visible from the anterior wall to the lateral wall of the left ventricle.

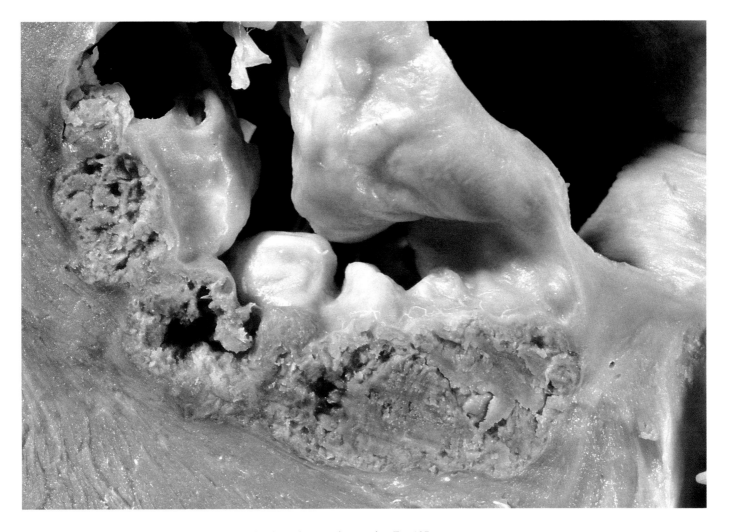

FIG. 128 Magnified view of the mitral valve annulus from the case discussed in Fig. 127. This shows the aggregated calcified deposits directly beneath the mitral valve with partial extension into the myocardium.

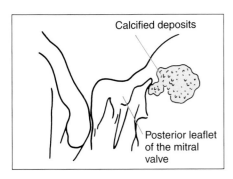

FIG. 129 View of the mitral valve on the long axis containing both the mitral and aortic valves (cardiac weight 820 g) in a 37-year-old man. Although a heart murmur was detected when the patient was in elementary school, he received no treatment. At age 30, he was diagnosed with both aortic and mitral insufficiency. Five and one-half years previously, the patient developed exertional dyspnea and atrial fibrillation. Five years previously, the patient underwent replacement of the aortic valve and a mitral commissurotomy. About 10 months before death, he again developed symptoms of exertional dyspnea. Echocardiography at that time showed sclerosis of the prosthetic valve and aortic regurgitation. Nineteen days before death, the patient underwent another aortic valve replacement; however, he developed multiorgan failure and death ensued. The leaflets of the mitral valve demonstrate marked fibrotic thickening. The chordae tendineae are fused and shortened. An aggregation of calcified deposits is seen just beneath the annulus.

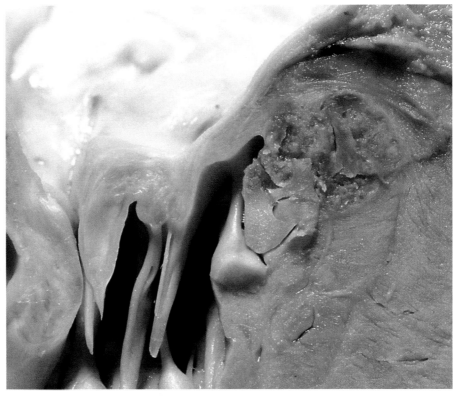

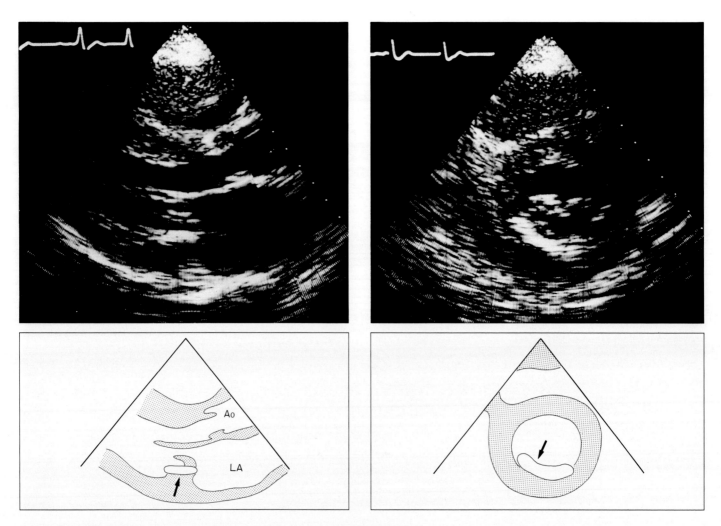

FIG. 130 (Left) Cross-sectional echocardiography on the long axis showing echoes with enhanced luminance of the mitral valve annulus near the posterior leaflet (arrow). Annular calcification is also present. (Right) Cross-sectional echocardiography along the short axis reveals calcification along the posterior aspect of the valve annulus (arrow). (Ao, aorta; LA, left atrium.)

Nonbacterial Thrombotic Endocarditis

Nonbacterial thrombotic endocarditis differs from infectious endocarditis in that no bacteria are present in the vegetations. Thus, there is a smooth outward appearance. The lesions primarily consist of platelets mixed with fibrin. Although lesions develop on the closed margins of the same valves commonly involved in rheumatic fever, the lesions are larger than those seen in rheumatic fever, and there is no valve destruction.

The mitral valve is most often affected, followed by the aortic valve, and then the tricuspid valve. Involvement of more than one valve is not uncommon.

The pathogenesis of nonbacterial thrombotic endocarditis has not been elucidated. Nevertheless, since this condition is often seen in association with mucin-producing malignant tumors and disseminated intravascular coagulation (DIC), it is thought to be related to abnormalities of blood coagulation. Because the disorder is sometimes seen in the terminal stages of serious illnesses, it is also called *marantic thrombus*. The clinical importance of this condition arises from its potential as a source of emboli.

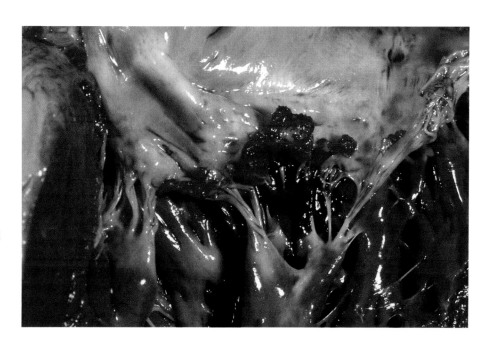

FIG. 131 View of the mitral valve after dissection of the lateral wall of the left ventricle (cardiac weight 490 g) of a 71-year-old man. At age 61, an arrhythmia and hypertension were detected. One month previously, right hemiplegia developed and the patient was hospitalized. During hospitalization the patient developed bloody stools and DIC and subsequently died. Abdominal echocardiography had indicated a tumor in the gallbladder. Autopsy showed carcinoma of the gallbladder (moderately differentiated adenocarcinoma). The presence of aggregated and shelf-like thrombotic vegetations extending over the anterior and posterior leaflets along the closed margins near the posterior commissure is shown.

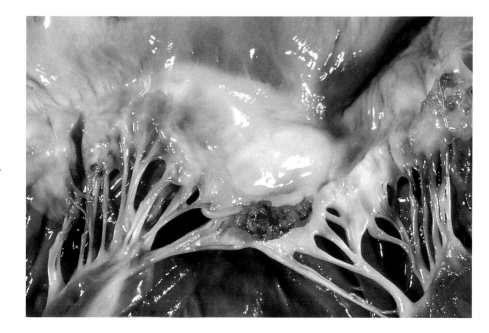

FIG. 132 View of the mitral valve of an 83-year-old man after dissection of the posterior wall of the left ventricle (cardiac weight 350 g). Previously, the patient had been generally well without history of any serious illnesses, but at age 80, he developed right-sided weakness and dementia. Chest radiographs yielded abnormal findings. During further diagnostic evaluation, the patient developed aspiration pneumonia and subsequently died. Autopsy showed small cell carcinoma in the right lung. Shelf-like thrombotic vegetations along the closed margins near the posterior commissure and the anterior leaflet are shown. The valve leaflets demonstrate age-related yellowish plaques and thickening of the closed margin.

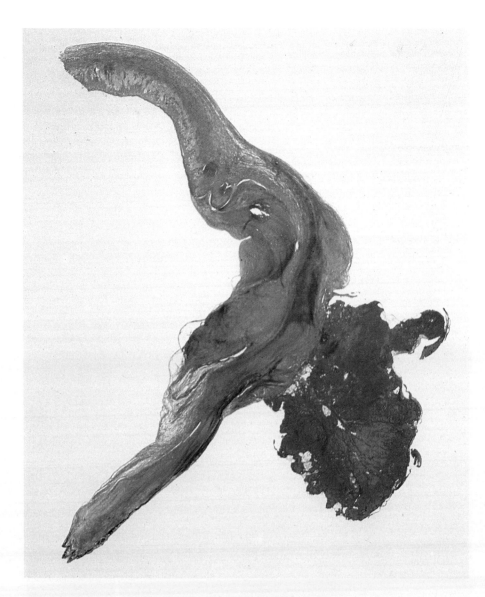

FIG. 133 Tissue section of the mitral valve anterior leaflet from the case discussed in Fig. 132. This reveals a thrombus near the closed margin. Rupture of the elastic fibers (black-violet area) is seen at the base of the leaflet. There is no evidence of neutrophilic infiltration or bacteria. (Elastica-HE stain, × 10.)

III
Aortic Valvular Disease

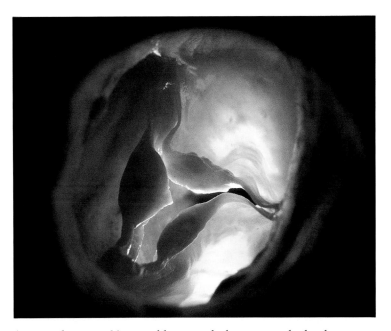

Aortic valve in an 80-year-old man with rheumatic valvular disease. The valve leaflets show fibrotic thickening and the commissures are mildly fused.

Rheumatic Valvular Disease

Most cases of rheumatic valvular disease in the aortic valve develop in combination with involvement of the mitral valve. Rheumatic mitral valvular disease is predominant in women, in contrast to aortic valvular disease, which is more frequently seen in men. Because of the anatomic position of the aortic valve and the regions affected, there are almost no instances of isolated stenosis or isolated insufficiency; most cases show a combination of both.

There are two basic pathophysiologic mechanisms in rheumatic aortic valvular disease: (1) fusion of the commissures, that is, adhesions of the semilunar valve in association with restriction of valve opening and (2) fibrosis of the semilunar valve itself. The former mechanism plays a role in stenosis, while the latter results in thickening and shortening of the valvular velum, contributing to regurgitation.

Aortic Stenosis and Insufficiency (Regurgitation)

Congenital aortic valvular disease is frequently associated with pure valvular stenosis, whereas rheumatic fever causes isolated stenosis in no more than 2% to 3% of cases. Adhesions of the commissures are one basic pathophysiologic factor in the rheumatic inflammatory process. This, plus the additional factor of valve thickening due to fibrosis, combine to alter the valvular structure. The area of the aortic valve orifice in adults is 2.5 to 3.5 cm^2. In mild stenosis with the valve orifice area reduced to 50% of normal, a systolic pressure gradient gradually develops between the left ventricle and the aorta. If this area is reduced to 1.0 cm^2, a moderate degree of obstruction results. A reduction in area to 0.5 cm^2 produces severe obstruction, and the normal balance can no longer be maintained between oxygen delivery by the coronary arteries and the workload of the left ventricle.

If contrast medium is injected just above the aortic valve, diagnostic imaging will depict regurgitation toward the left ventricle during diastole and a protruding dome-like filling defect toward the aorta during systole. If there is sclerosis of the valve, the dome formation becomes irregular and protrusion is less. Severe valve thickening is visible as hypertranslucency. Regurgitation is assessed by the width of the jet, the amount of contrast medium moving into the apex, and the degree of blushing. A narrow jet indicates little regurgitation; a wide jet represents severe regurgitation.

Echocardiography shows thickening, enhanced luminance, and restricted opening of the aortic valve, along with fusion of the commissures. If regurgitation is present, it will produce visible dilation of the left ventricular cavity and evidence of vibration in the anterior leaflet of the mitral valve and in the interventricular septum. Severe stenosis produces hypertrophy of the interventricular septum and left ventricular wall.

Doppler techniques allow the use of a continuous-wave Doppler method, with approach from the cardiac apex, suprasternal space, or right edge of the sternum, to record maximum flow velocity through the aortic valve orifice during systole. From this, the pressure gradient is calculated across the aortic valve using a simplified Bernoulli's method. The pressure gradient of the aortic valve using this Doppler method is expressed as the *maximum pressure gradient*. There is some difference between this and the *peak to peak* pressure gradient measured by catheter methods. In general, the maximum pressure gradient is larger with Doppler techniques.

In rheumatic aortic valvular disease, both stenosis and insufficiency are present in a large percentage of cases. The severity of each may vary, but the presence of even a mild second condition can have an overall adverse clinical effect. For example, aortic stenosis limits the increase of stroke volume that is available to compensate for the regurgitation produced by valvular insufficiency. In such cases, even though aortic regurgitation may not be severe when assessed by methods such as cardiac catheterization, early surgical intervention must be considered; such surgery almost always involves valve replacement. After thoroughly removing any calcifications from the annulus of the original valve, a prosthetic heart valve is implanted. In cases of combined valvular disease in which mitral valvular disease predominates, a commissurotomy or debridement (or both) may be performed for milder lesions.

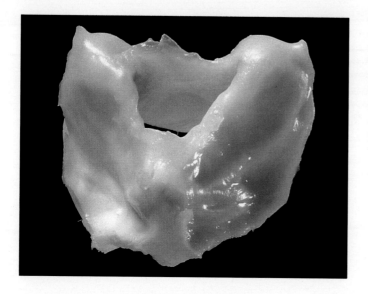

FIG. 134 Resected aortic valve. The patient was a 61-year-old woman. At age 43, she developed exertional dyspnea and was diagnosed with valvular disease. Approximately 2.5 years previously, right homonymous hemianopsia developed but subsequently improved. One and one-half years previously, the patient began to experience chest pain when walking. One year previously, she was diagnosed with aortic stenosis and insufficiency, mitral stenosis and insufficiency, and atrial fibrillation. The aortic valve was replaced, and a commissurotomy of the mitral valve was performed. Marked fibrotic thickening of the valve leaflets and fusion of the commissures are shown.

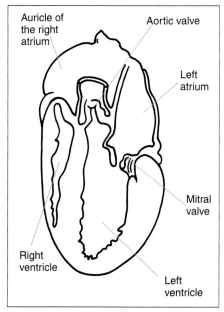

Auricle of
the right
atrium

Aortic valve

Left
atrium

Mitral
valve

Right
ventricle

Left
ventricle

FIG. 135 A longitudinal cross-section, including the mitral and aortic valves (cardiac
weight 560 g), of a 40-year-old man. At age
10, he contracted rheumatic fever, and at age
32, a heart murmur was detected. Beginning at
age 35, the patient developed exertional dyspnea. About 2 months before death, there was
the onset of fever and symptoms of heart failure. Antibiotics were given and surgery was
scheduled, but the patient developed an
arrhythmia and subsequently died. Fibrotic
thickening of the leaflets of the mitral valve is
shown. The chordae tendineae are shortened,
and the spaces between them have disap-
peared. The mitral valve is funnel-shaped, and
there is left ventricular dilation and hypertrophy of the wall. The aortic valve also shows
marked fibrotic thickening, as well as calcified
deposits and fusion of the commissures.

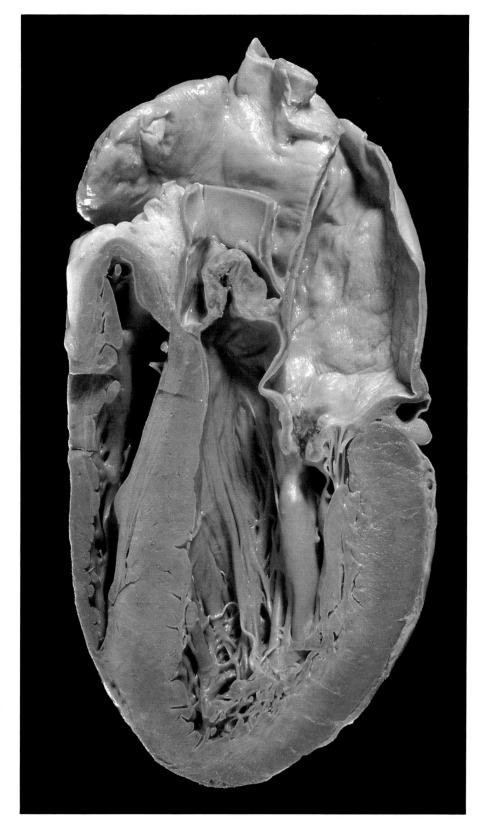

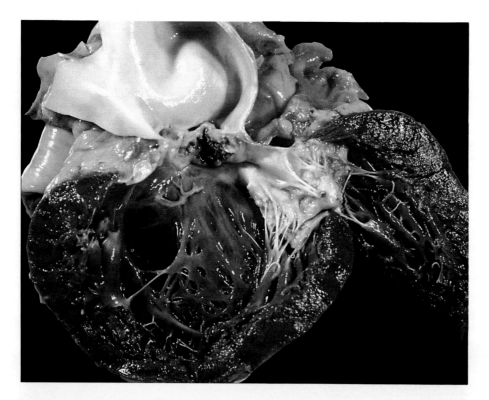

FIG. 136 View of the left ventricular outflow tract of a 63-year-old woman after dissection of the anterior and posterior walls of the left ventricle (cardiac weight 640 g). She had contracted rheumatic fever while in elementary school. Beginning at age 52, the patient developed exertional dyspnea. She was diagnosed with combined valvular disease and received treatment by her local physician. One month before death her symptoms worsened. One day before death, she was hospitalized on an emergency basis because of anasarca and dehydration. She then developed atrial fibrillation and died. Fibrotic thickening, calcified deposits, ulcer formation, and thrombi on the aortic valve are shown. The left ventricle is dilated. A jet lesion (endocardial pocket) due to regurgitation is visible in the endocardium just below the aortic valve. The aorta is dilated.

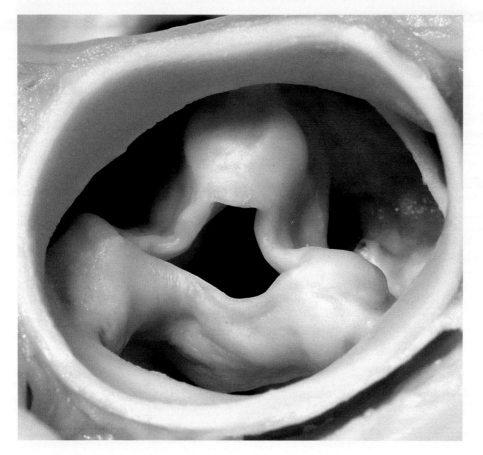

FIG. 137 View from the aortic side of the aortic valve (cardiac weight 580 g) of a 54-year-old woman. At age 24, valvular disease was diagnosed. One and one-half years previously, the patient developed exertional dyspnea and generalized fatigue, followed 3 months previously by the onset of irregular palpitations. The patient was hospitalized 2 months previously for treatment of heart failure and more detailed clinical evaluation. Although she received treatment, her condition gradually worsened and she subsequently died. Marked fibrotic thickening of the valve leaflets and fusion of the commissures are seen. The valvular orifice has a fish-mouth appearance.

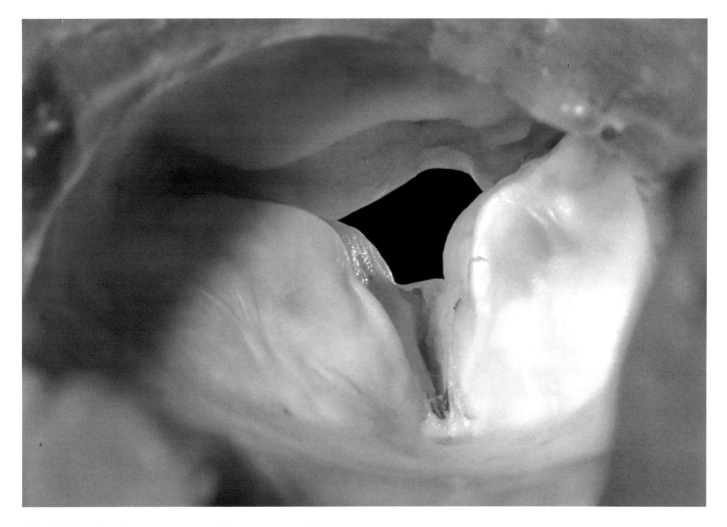

FIG. 138 View from the ventricular side of the aortic valve of the case discussed in Fig. 137. The valve leaflets exhibit fibrotic thickening and fusion of the commissures. The valvular orifice has a fish-mouth appearance.

FIG. 139 View from the ventricular side of the aortic valve (cardiac weight 460 g) of a 62-year-old man. At age 40, he developed symptoms of heart failure, followed several years before death by the onset of cough with hemoptysis and 2 years previously by dyspnea and orthopnea. The patient was diagnosed with aortic stenosis and insufficiency, mitral stenosis and insufficiency, and pulmonary hypertension. Surgery was recommended, but the patient declined. Subsequent gradual worsening of heart failure was followed by death. Fibrotic thickening of the valve leaflets, rough surfaces, and large brownish calcified deposits are seen. The commissures are fused, and Lambl's excrescences (projections) are visible.

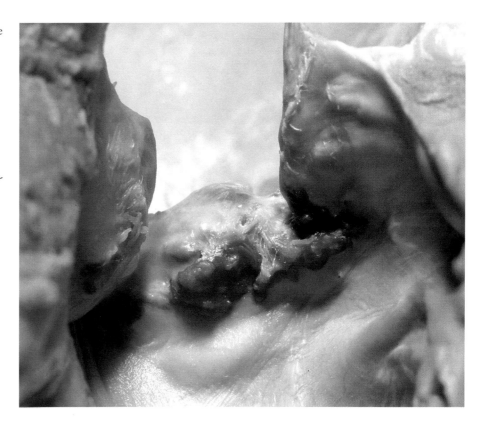

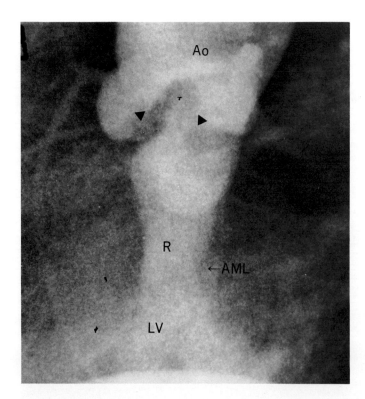

FIG. 140 Aortic angiography (lateral view) shows marked thickening of the valve leaflets (black arrow) and regurgitation into the left ventricle. (Ao, aorta; AML, anterior mitral leaflet; LV, left ventricle; R, regurgitation.)

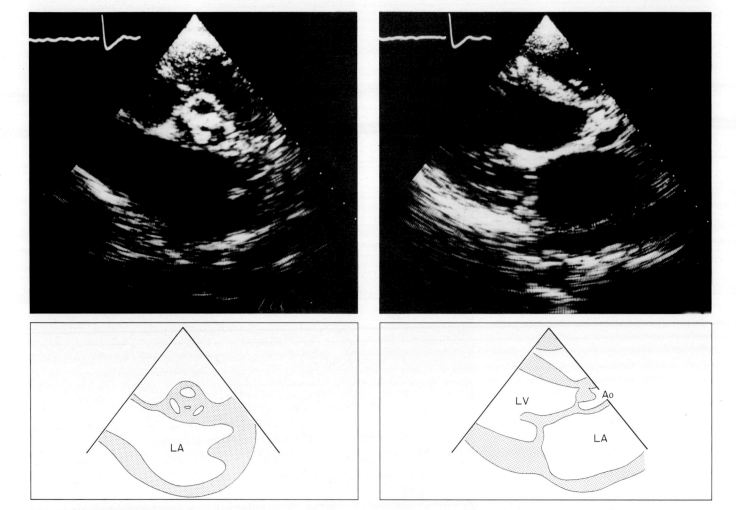

FIG. 141 Echocardiography. (Left) Cross-sectional echocardiography along the short axis at the level of the aortic valve shows a thickened aortic valve with three cusps visible. Even during systole this valve barely opens. (Right) Cross-sectional echocardiography along the long axis reveals thickening of the aortic valve. This patient also had concomitant mitral valvular disease. (Ao, aorta; LA, left atrium; LV, left ventricle.)

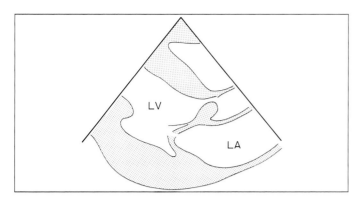

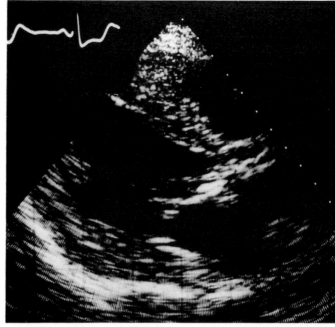

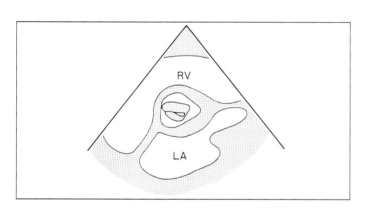

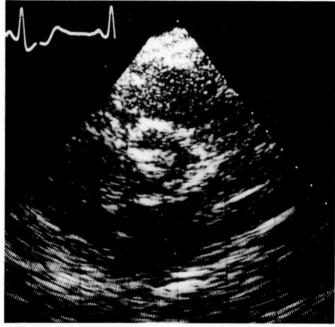

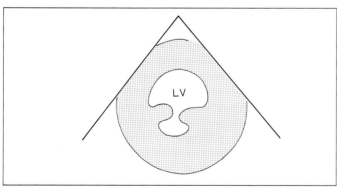

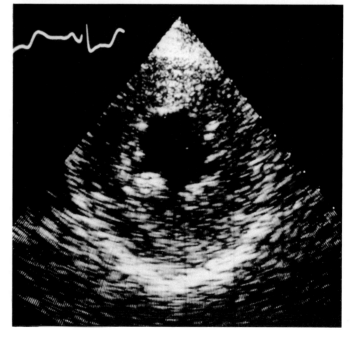

FIG. 142 (Top) Cross-sectional echocardiography along the long axis shows thickening of the aortic valve. (Middle) Cross-sectional echocardiography along the short axis during mid-systole (aortic valve level) shows poor valve opening. The valve appears bivalvular because of adhesions. (Bottom) Short axis cross-sectional echocardiography at the level of the papillary muscles demonstrates homogeneous hypertrophy of the interventricular septum and free wall. (LA, left atrium; LV, left ventricle; RV, right ventricle.)

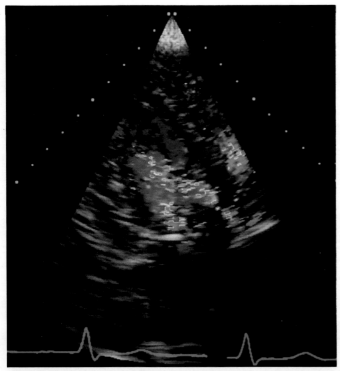

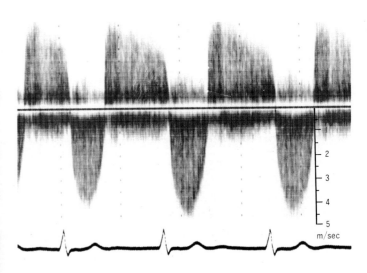

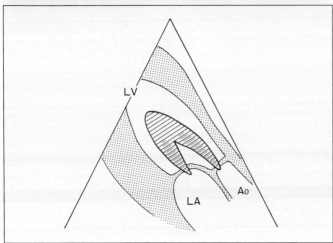

FIG. 143 Doppler imaging. (Left) Cross-sectional imaging along the long axis of the left ventricle during diastole records a reddish, jet-like, aortic valve regurgitant signal from the valve orifice into the left ventricle. In the center of the left ventricle, there is a confluence with incoming blood flow of the mitral valve. (Right) A continuous-wave Doppler method, apical approach, was used to record blood flow in aortic stenosis during systole and the regurgitant blood flow signal during diastole. Flow velocity in aortic stenosis is approximately 4.5 m/sec. The pressure gradient across the aortic valvular orifice obtained by the simplified Bernoulli's equation ($p = 4V^2$ [p, pressure gradient across the valve orifice; V, maximum flow velocity]) is approximately 80 mmHg. (Ao, aorta; LA, left atrium; LV, left ventricle.)

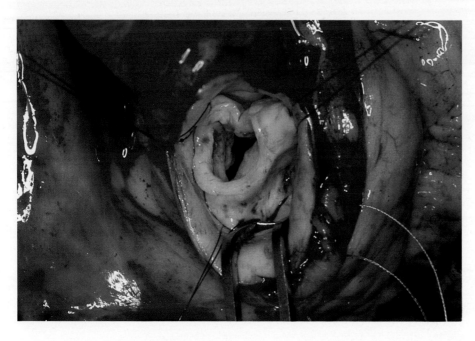

FIG. 144 Intraoperative photograph. There is fusion of the commissures and marked valve thickening. The entire valve has a fish-mouth appearance.

Aortic Insufficiency (Regurgitation)

Vegetations develop on the closed margins of the valve as a result of inflammatory tissue and thrombus formation. There is organization of inflammatory exudates on the valvular velum, with resultant contraction, thickening, deformation, and shortening. This leads to a triangular defect in the center of the valve during diastole. The free margins of the valve are thickened and usually invaginate toward the sinus. Such changes are exacerbated by further secondary degenerative changes, most commonly due to recurrent rheumatic fever, or in some cases, to atherosclerosis or calcification.

Diagnostic aortic angiography shows no dome formation of the aortic valve. Regurgitation is evaluated by the width of the regurgitant jet, the amount of contrast medium reaching the apex, and the degree of blushing. When the jet width is narrow, there is little regurgitation; when the jet width is wide, there is severe regurgitation. Evaluation is based on a three- or four-stage scale.

With Doppler techniques, using an apical or parasternal approach, the region from the aortic valve orifice to within the left ventricle is evaluated during diastole. With an apical approach, the maximum recorded area of regurgitation is measured. Then, the degree of regurgitation is classified on a four-stage scale. It is necessary to thoroughly distinguish and separate this component of regurgitation from the blood flowing through the mitral valve orifice into the left ventricle. It is possible to evaluate the site of regurgitation by using short-axis cross-sectional views of the aortic valve orifice to record the location of regurgitation.

In aortic regurgitation, thickening of the valve leaflets is mild. However, there is often shortening of the leaflets. Surgical intervention consists of valve replacement.

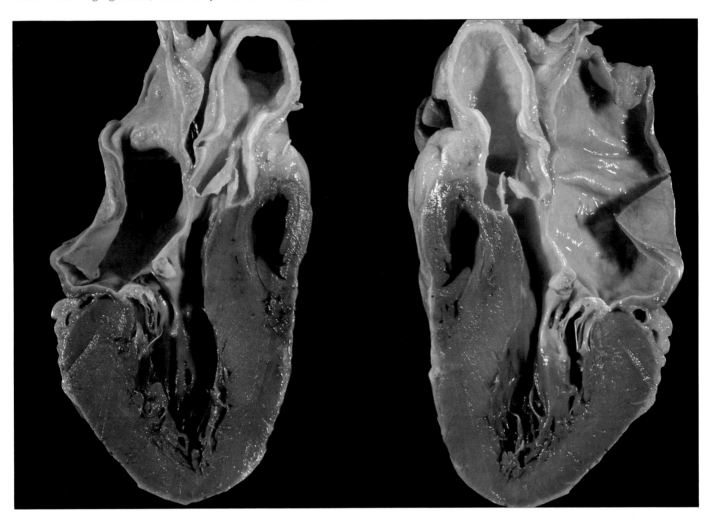

FIG. 145 Long-axis cross-sectional view of the heart, including the mitral and aortic valves (cardiac weight 600 g), of a 69-year-old man. At age 13, he contracted rheumatic fever, and a heart murmur was detected. One and one-half years previously, the patient noticed swelling in his lower extremities. Five days before death, atrial fibrillation was seen on electrocardiogram and the patient was hospitalized for detailed studies. One day before death, he developed abdominal pain and symptoms compatible with an ileus. Abdominal angiography showed multiple defects in the mesenteric artery. Although emergency surgery was performed, the procedure was stopped at the point of exploratory laparotomy because of extensive necrosis. Subsequently the patient died. Fibrotic thickening of the mitral valve leaflets, fusion and shortening of the chordae tendineae, and left ventricular hypertrophy are shown. There is mild fibrotic thickening of the aortic valve with slight elongation.

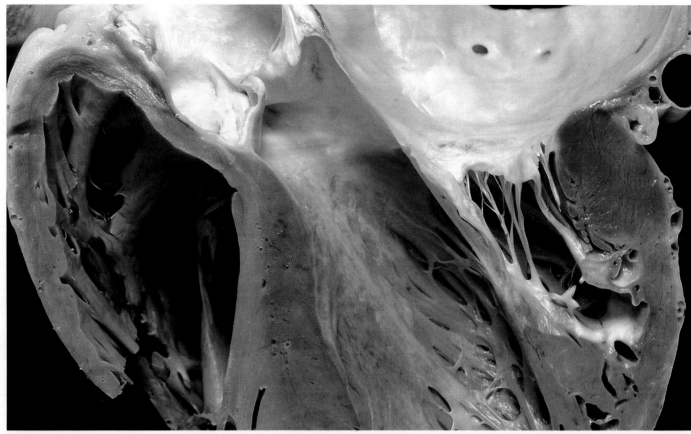

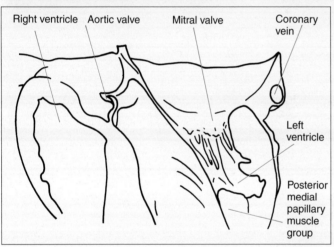

Right ventricle | Aortic valve | Mitral valve | Coronary vein

Left ventricle

Posterior medial papillary muscle group

FIG. 146 Long-axis cross-sectional view that includes the mitral and aortic valves (cardiac weight 650 g) of the case discussed in Fig. 48. The leaflets of the mitral and aortic valves exhibit marked fibrotic thickening and fusion of the commissures. The chordae tendineae are fused and fibrotic. Fibrotic thickening of the endocardium is present. There is visible thinning of the free wall of the left ventricle and an increase in fibrotic tissue.

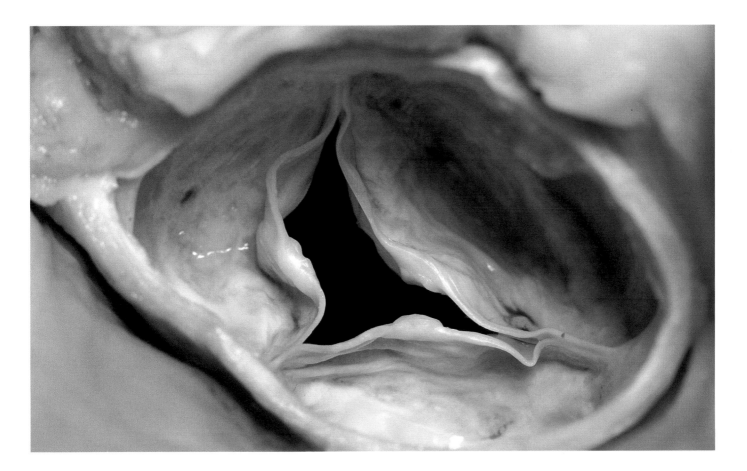

FIG. 147 View from the aortic side of the aortic valve of the case discussed in Fig. 146. There is mild fibrotic thickening of the leaflets of the aortic valve and slight fusion of the commissures. The valvular ring is dilated and the leaflets are elongated. Age-related changes such as xanthomas of the valve leaflets and calcified deposits of the aorta are visible.

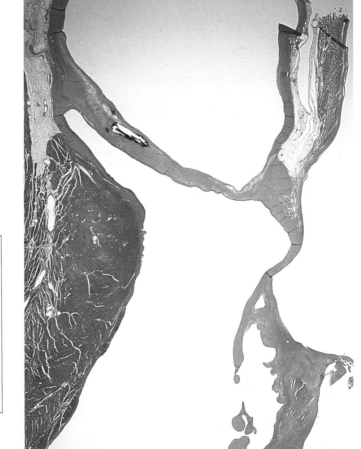

Left atrial wall

Aortic valve

Mitral valve

FIG. 148 Tissue section image of the aortic and mitral valves of the case discussed in Fig. 146. The leaflets of the aortic valve show fibrotic thickening and calcified deposits. The leaflets of the mitral valve also exhibit marked fibrotic thickening.

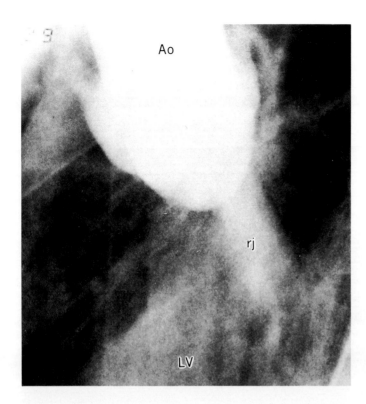

FIG. 149 Aortic angiography (60-degree left anterior oblique). A regurgitant jet has developed from between the left coronary cusp and the noncoronary cusp. A moderate degree of regurgitation is present. (Ao, aorta; LV, left ventricle; rj, regurgitant jet.)

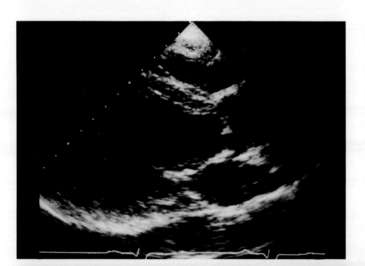

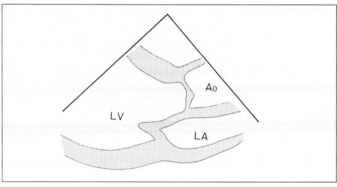

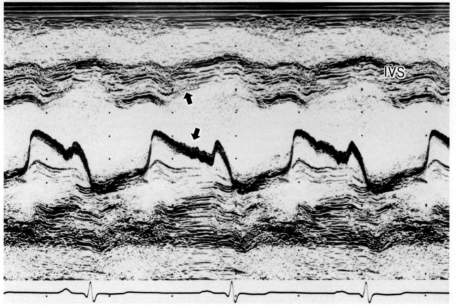

FIG. 150 (Top) Cross-sectional echocardiography along the long axis shows thickening of the aortic valve. Left ventricular dilation has developed due to aortic regurgitation. (Bottom) M-mode echocardiography shows a small amount of vibration (arrow) of the anterior leaflet of the mitral valve and the interventricular septum, also due to aortic regurgitation. (Ao, aorta; IVS, interventricular septum; LA, left atrium; LV, left ventricle.)

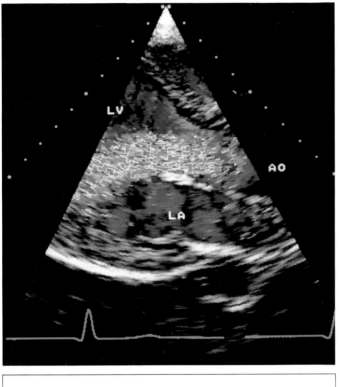

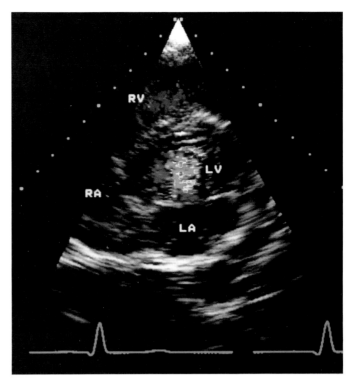

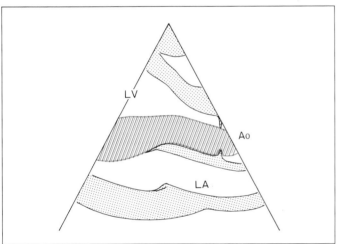

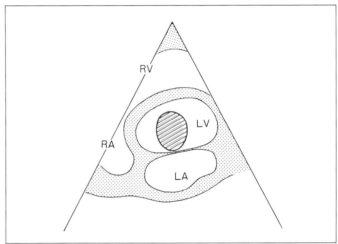

FIG. 151 Doppler imaging. (Left) Parasternal cross-sectional imaging through the long axis of the left ventricle recorded a wide regurgitant signal from the aortic valve during systole within the left ventricle from the aortic valve orifice along the anterior leaflet of the mitral valve. The degree of regurgitation was considered severe based on the width of this regurgitant signal. (Right) Cross-sectional imaging on the short axis of the left ventricular outflow tract recorded a circular regurgitant signal during diastole. This was thought to be the short-axis cross section of the aortic regurgitant jet. (Ao, aorta; LA, left atrium; LV, left ventricle; RA, right atrium; RV, right ventricle.)

FIG. 152 Intraoperative photograph showing thickening of the valve margins and curling. There is very mild fusion of the commissures but no hemodynamically significant stenosis.

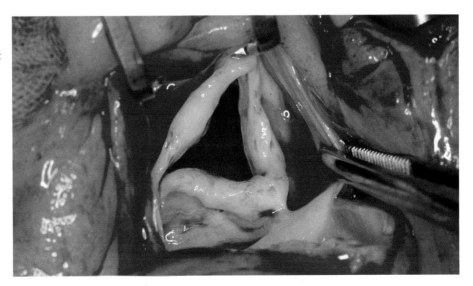

Congenital Bicuspid Valve

Congenital bicuspid valve is an important condition that can produce stenosis involving the aortic valve alone. Particularly in cases of isolated calcified aortic stenosis in elderly patients, a congenital bicuspid valve is a more likely etiology than rheumatic valvular disease. In nonrheumatic aortic stenosis, it is said that 60% of patients younger than age 15 have a unicuspid valve and a single commissure, 60% of patients age 15 to 65 have a bicuspid valve, and 90% of patients older than age 65 have a tricuspid valve. In addition to being bicuspid, a congenital bicuspid valve usually shows a morphologically characteristic fibrous structure (raphe) connecting one of the valve leaflets to the medial wall of the aorta. The most important complication of congenital bicuspid valves is stenosis, followed by complications of insufficiency and infectious endocarditis.

Stenosis and Insufficiency (Regurgitation)

Angiography of the ascending aorta shows the bulging of only two leaflets of the aortic valve. These leaflets may be equal or unequal in size. In stenosis, dome formation is seen during systole; if valvular insufficiency is present, regurgitation is seen during diastole.

In echocardiography, it is necessary to use cross-sectional echocardiography to verify that the aortic valve has two leaflets. Generally the leaflet in the anterior position is larger. The valve often resembles a tricuspid valve because of the presence of the raphe, so care is required. When severe calcification is present, it can be difficult to determine whether the valve is truly bicuspid. M-mode echocardiography shows that the valve does not close at the center of the aorta, but deviates toward the anterior or posterior wall. If stenosis is severe, left ventricular wall hypertrophy is usually present. Valvular insufficiency produces visible vibration of the interventricular septum and the anterior leaflet of the mitral valve, secondary to regurgitation. There will also be left ventricular dilation.

Surgical intervention involves valve replacement except in infants. There are instances in which the valvular annulus itself is narrow and a prosthetic valve of adequate size cannot be used. Thus, in some cases the annulus is enlarged with a patch. Calcification of the valve ring is often more severe than in rheumatic valvular disease.

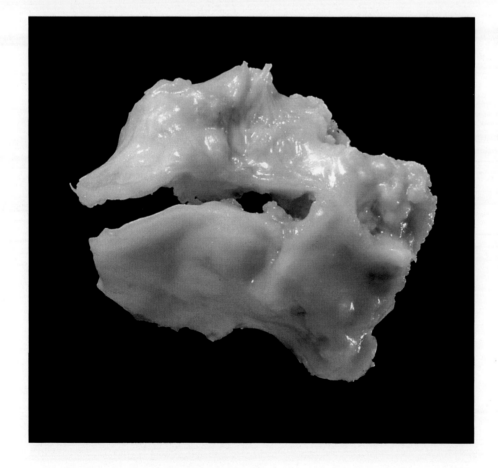

FIG. 153 View from the aortic side of a resected aortic valve. There is thickening of the valve leaflets, and prominent calcified deposits are visible. The raphe is not clearly visible.

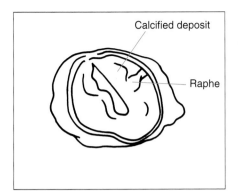

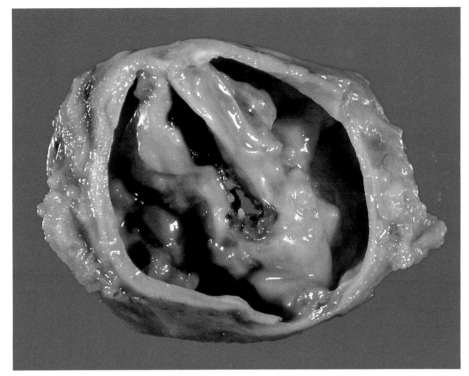

FIG. 154 View from the aortic side after dissection of a bicuspid aortic valve and aorta (cardiac weight 800 g). This is the case of a 61-year-old man who developed acute nephritis at age 9. At age 58, he was diagnosed with cardiomegaly, and hemodialysis was initiated. Two months previously, he developed symptoms of heart failure. Ten days before death, he began having episodes of chest pain. The patient was diagnosed by Doppler echocardiography as having both aortic stenosis and insufficiency. Surgery was scheduled, but the patient experienced an episode of chest pain during defecation, lost consciousness, and subsequently died. Fibrotic thickening of the valve leaflets with marked calcified deposits is shown. There is fusion of the commissures. A raphe is present on the larger valve leaflet.

FIG. 155 View from the aortic side of an aortic valve (cardiac weight 700 g) of a 72-year-old woman. At age 55, she was diagnosed with valvular heart disease. At age 68, she was diagnosed with both aortic stenosis and insufficiency, and conservative medical therapy was prescribed. Two months before death, the patient contracted an upper respiratory infection and experienced progressive worsening of heart failure. She subsequently died. The two leaflets in the aortic valve are shown. There is fibrotic thickening of the leaflets and calcified deposits. The valve orifice has a slit-like appearance. A raphe is seen on the larger valve leaflet.

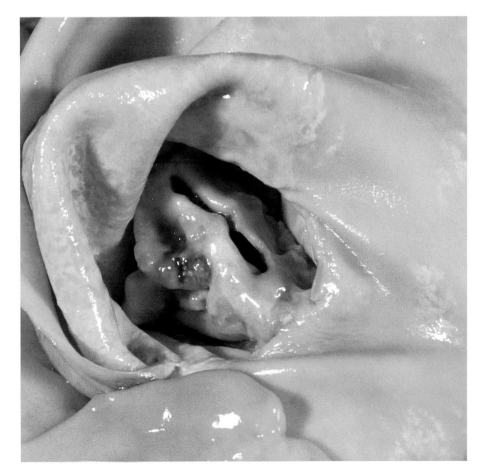

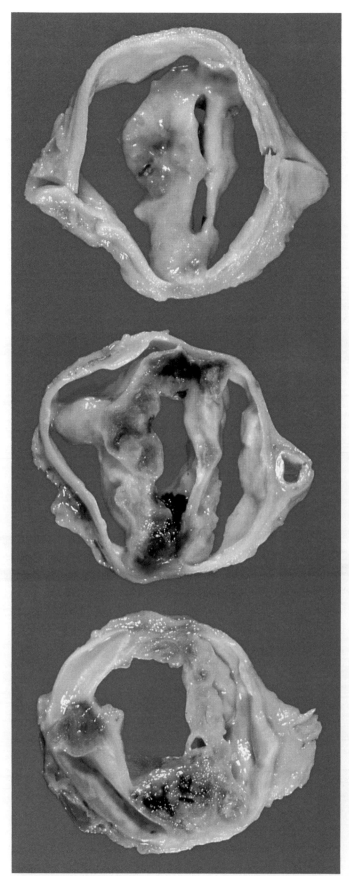

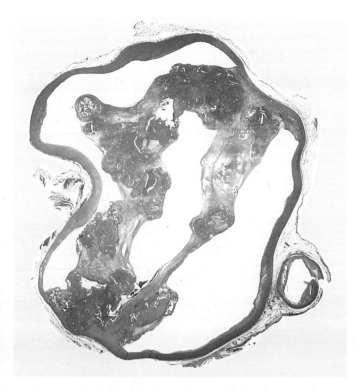

FIG. 157 Tissue section of the congenital bicuspid valve of the case discussed in Fig. 155 showing bilateral openings of the coronary arteries. Calcification is pronounced, and the raphe is visible. (HE stain.)

FIG. 156 Round sections of the aortic valve of the case discussed in Fig. 155, following resection from the heart and decalcification. The slit-like valvular orifice is prominent. A raphe is visible in the middle section. There is marked calcification.

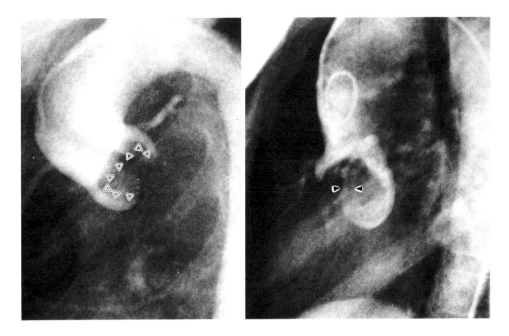

FIG. 158 Angiographic findings in congenital aortic stenosis. The aortic valve is bicuspid. (Left) Tangential view of the aortic valve along a cephalad axis (shallow left anterior oblique) shows "negative" dome formation. (Right) Aortic valve orifice (orifice view). The number of valve leaflets is clearly depicted, and there is visible fusion of the commissures. (Black arrow, juncture of right and left coronary cusps.)

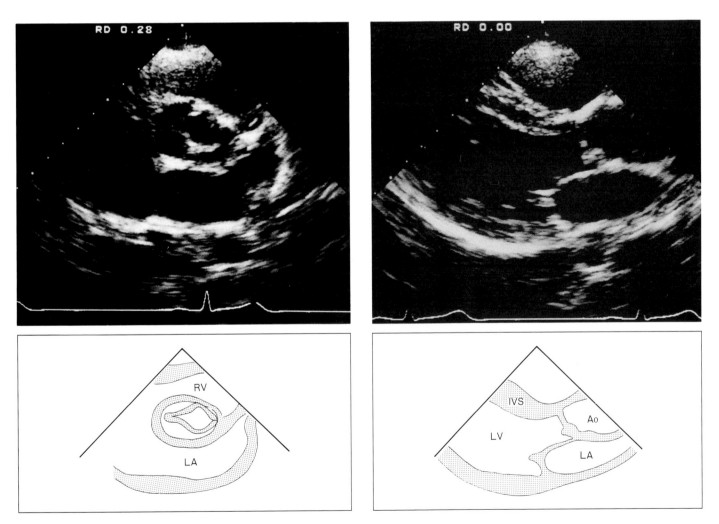

FIG. 159 (Left) Cross-sectional echocardiography along the short axis demonstrates that the aortic valve is bicuspid. Medial valve opening is somewhat poor. (Right) Cross-sectional echocardiography along the long axis shows that the dorsal aspect of the aortic valve protrudes slightly toward the left ventricle. Since the degree of stenosis is mild, there is no hypertrophy of the left ventricular wall. (Ao, aorta; IVS, interventricular septum; LA, left atrium; LV, left ventricle; RV, right ventricle.)

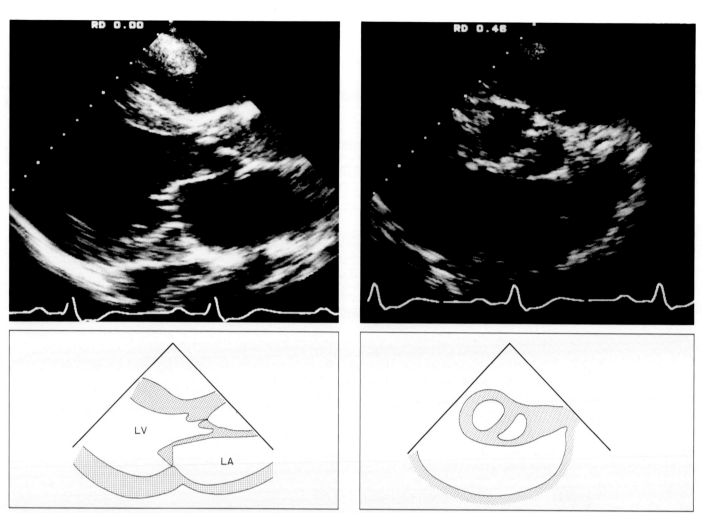

FIG. 160 (Left) Cross-sectional echocardiography along the long axis shows thickening of the aortic valve. Combined stenosis and insufficiency is suspected on the basis of the hypertrophic ventricular wall and dilated left ventricular cavity. (Right) Cross-sectional echocardiography along the short axis at the level of the aortic valve shows thickening of the bicuspid valve. The right upper part of the valve is slightly enlarged. (LA, left atrium; LV, left ventricle.)

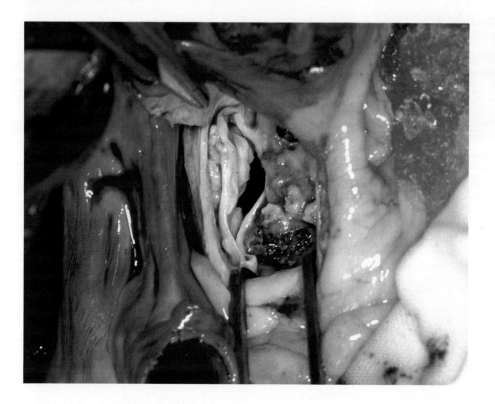

FIG. 161 Intraoperative photograph showing the shape of the right and left cusps. Although there is no fusion of the commissures, prominent calcification is visible and the opening is slit-shaped.

Insufficiency (Regurgitation)

Insufficiency (regurgitation) is often complicated by infectious endocarditis. Please refer to the previous section regarding diagnostic imaging and echocardiography. Surgical intervention involves valve replacement.

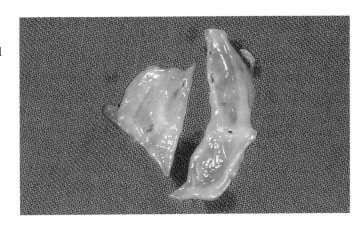

FIG. 162 Resected bicuspid aortic valve. The patient was a 38-year-old man. He was healthy at birth and participated in athletics as a student. Eight months previously, a heart murmur was detected during a medical examination. The diagnosis was aortic insufficiency as a result of a bicuspid aortic valve. The patient underwent surgical replacement of the aortic valve. Some thickening and folding of the valve margin of the larger valve leaflet, as well as a small perforation is seen. A raphe is also present.

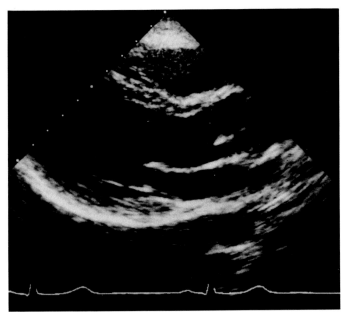

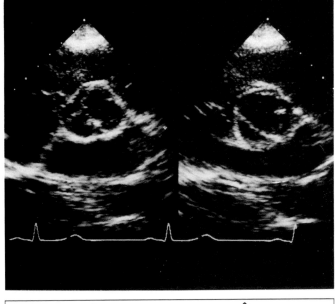

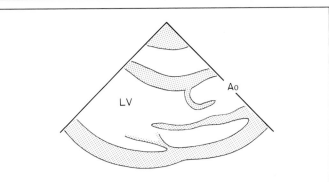

FIG. 163 (Left) Cross-sectional echocardiography along the long axis reveals prolapse of the anterior part of the valve into the left ventricle. (Right) Cross-sectional echocardiography along the short axis (right side, systole; left side, diastole) shows the larger anterior and the smaller posterior leaflets of the valve. There is a raphe on the medial aspect of the anterior leaflet. (Ao, aorta; LA, left atrium; LV, left ventricle; RA, right atrium; RV, right ventricle.)

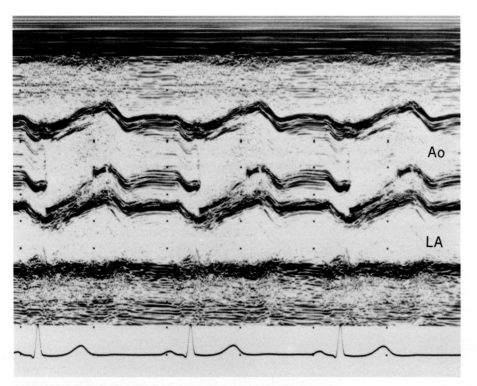

Ao

LA

FIG. 164 M-mode echocardiography of the case discussed in Fig. 163.
Valve closure has shifted dorsally from the center of the aorta. (Ao,
aorta; LA, left atrium.)

Infectious Endocarditis

The incidence of infectious endocarditis involving the aortic valve alone is 60%. This incidence is low in comparison with an 80% incidence of isolated involvement of the mitral valve. The incidence of combined involvement of the aortic and mitral valves is said to be 40%. Infectious endocarditis accompanied by aortic insufficiency occurs most frequently at the aortic valve on the side opening into the left ventricle, and next most frequently involves the chordae tendineae of the anterior leaflet of the mitral valve.

Vegetations

When large vegetations adhere to the aortic valve, aortic angiography reveals thick filling defects of the valve leaflets. Echocardiography shows an abnormal aggregation of echoes in the left ventricle, mainly of the aortic valve. During systole, these echoes cross the aortic valve and sometimes enter into the aorta from the left ventricle.

Since fairly large vegetations may lead to embolic complications above the mitral valve, early valve replacement is recommended.

See Chapter 2 for a discussion of the pathologic and morphologic findings.

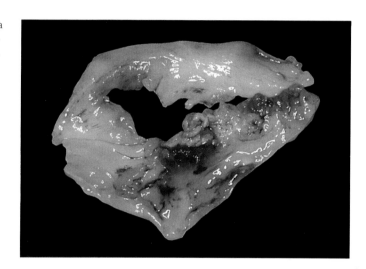

FIG. 165 View from the ventricular side of a resected aortic valve from a 27-year-old man. Two months previously, he began experiencing palpitations; 1 month previously, a heart murmur was detected. Echocardiography revealed vegetations of the aortic valve, and the patient was given antibiotics. Further enlargement of the vegetations led to replacement of the aortic valve. The aortic valve is bicuspid. Adherent thrombotic vegetations with a granular surface are visible near the closing margins of the valve, and there is marked destruction of the valve margins.

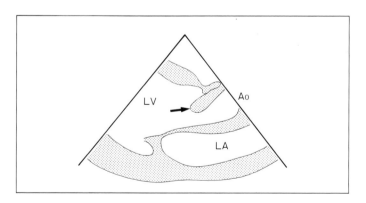

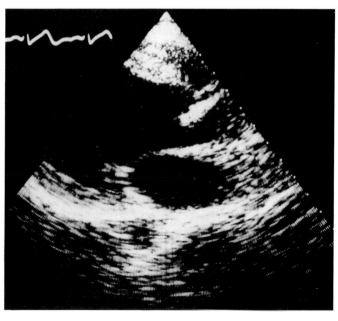

FIG. 166 Cross-sectional echocardiography along the long axis depicts vegetations on the aortic valve (arrow). (Ao, aorta; LA, left atrium; LV, left ventricle.)

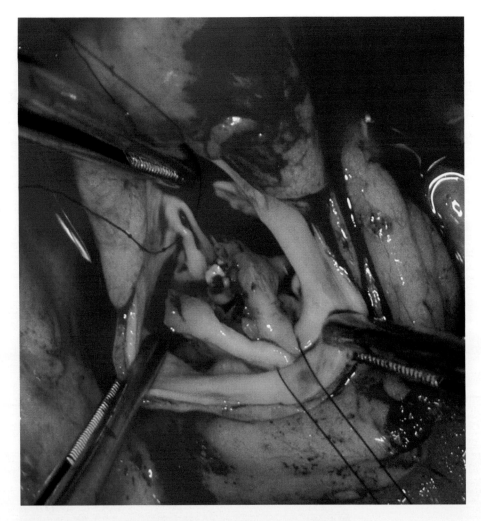

FIG. 167 Intraoperative photograph showing vegetations on the left coronary cusp. There are still characteristics of an active stage of infection.

Aneurysm and Perforation

According to Aschoff and colleagues, aneurysms of the mitral valve often protrude into the left atrium, while aneurysms of the aortic valve frequently protrude into the left ventricle.

Aortic angiography shows these aneurysms as knob-like shadows in the direction of the left ventricle. If a perforation develops in the aneurysm, regurgitation arises from this region toward the left ventricle.

Echocardiography reveals knob-like echoes of the aortic valve into the left ventricle, similar to echoes seen with mitral valve aneurysms. Where perforations are present, the valvular echo shows rupture.

Surgical intervention in the form of valvuloplasty can be difficult even during the healing phase. Unless the perforation is small, the valve is usually replaced.

For pathologic and morphologic findings, see Chapter 2.

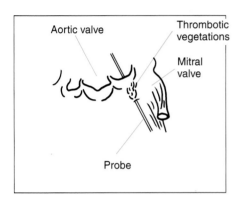

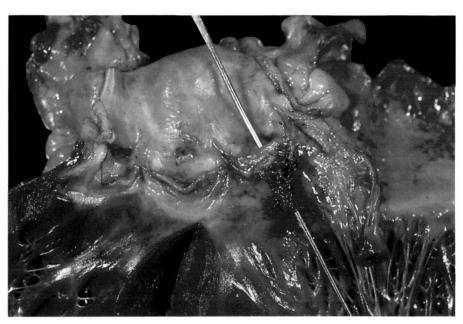

FIG. 168 View of the left ventricular outflow tract of a 26-year-old man. At age 16, a heart murmur was detected. About 1 month before death, the patient developed a persistent fever, edema of the lower extremities, and exertional dyspnea. The diagnosis was endocarditis; blood cultures showed group C *Streptococcus*. Although intensive antibiotic therapy was initiated, there was no improvement in the clinical findings, and surgery was scheduled. However, the patient died of a cerebral hemorrhage. Thrombotic vegetations on the noncoronary cusp of the aortic valve are shown. The probe demonstrates the presence of a perforation.

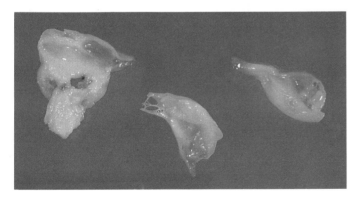

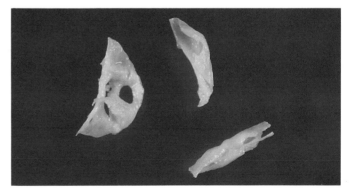

FIG. 169 Resected aortic valve from a 41-year-old woman. A heart murmur was detected at age 29. The patient had a persistent fever beginning three months previously; α-*Streptococcus* was isolated in blood cultures. Although intensive antibiotic therapy was given, there was no improvement, and surgery was performed. Doppler echocardiography showed a ventricular septal defect, aortic insufficiency, and vegetations on the aortic valve. A large perforation at the base of one valve leaflet is seen. There are also thrombotic vegetations in this region. A tissue section of these vegetations shows numerous gram-positive cocci.

FIG. 170 Resected aortic valve from a 38-year-old man. Hypertension and a heart murmur were detected in a medical examination at approximately age 23. One and one-half years previously, he began to experience generalized fatigue on mild exertion. Ten months previously, he began experiencing nocturnal dyspnea and chest pressure. Aortic insufficiency was diagnosed and the patient underwent aortic valve replacement. Several large perforations in one of the valve leaflets are seen. There are yellow-white opacities and thickening of the leaflet around these perforations.

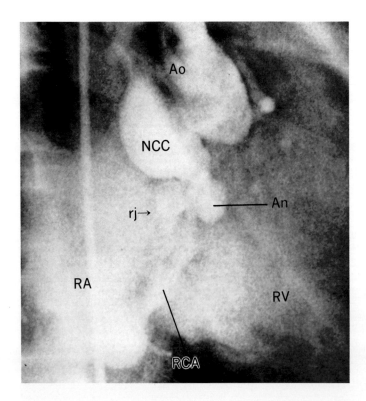

FIG. 171 A rare case in which an aneurysm of the right coronary cusp has perforated into the right atrium. Right anterior oblique view of an aortic angiogram, showing a jet of contrast medium into the right atrium from the ruptured perforation of the aneurysm in the noncoronary cusp. The right atrium is contrasted in comparison to the right ventricle. (An, aneurysm; Ao, aorta; NCC, noncoronary cusp; RA, right atrium; RCA, right coronary artery; rj, regurgitant jet; RV, right ventricle.)

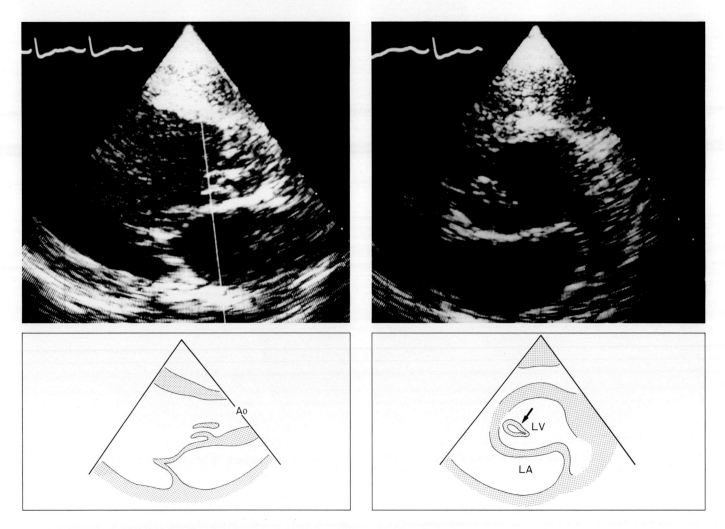

FIG. 172 (Left) Cross-sectional echocardiography along the long axis shows protrusion of the noncoronary cusp into the left ventricle, suggesting the presence of an aneurysm and vegetations of the aortic valve. There are also findings of left ventricular dilation. (Right) Cross-sectional echocardiography along the short axis reveals the site where the noncoronary cusp protrudes into the left ventricle (arrow). This may be the perforation of the aneurysm. (Ao, aorta; LA, left atrium; LV, left ventricle.)

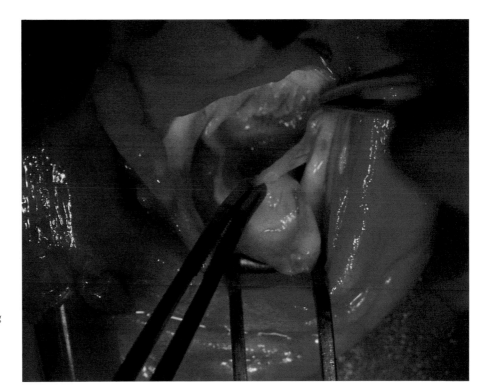

FIG. 173 Intraoperative photograph depicting a large aneurysm of the right coronary cusp protruding into the left ventricle. There is a perforation measuring several millimeters at the tip.

FIG. 174 Intraoperative photograph showing a perforation of the noncoronary cusp during the healing stage of inflammation.

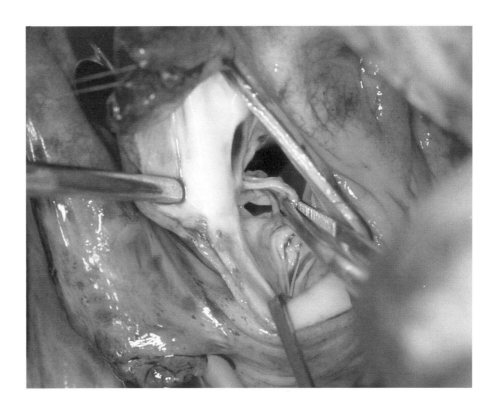

Aortic Annular Abscess

One fairly common complication of infectious endocarditis is valvular annular abscess, seen in 27% to 86% of cases at autopsy and in 10% to 20% of cases during surgery.

Annular abscesses most often involve the aortic valve. Autopsy cases in which these abscesses are present show a higher incidence of endocarditis, second degree (or greater) atrioventricular block, and valvular regurgitation than is seen in cases in which such abscesses are absent. Echocardiography detects abnormal cavities that are not generally seen in the periphery of the aortic valve annulus.

Reports have indicated that *Staphylococcus aureus* and *Pneumococcus* are frequently isolated as the causative organisms in these annular abscesses. However, results are not uniform in this regard.

In cases complicated by an abscess, although other sites of inflammation may improve with antibiotic administration, the abscess itself often remains. Rapid surgical intervention is therefore important. Surgery consists of complete excision of the abscess and resection of the infected tissues, followed by reconstruction of the aortic wall using a patch. A portion of a prosthetic heart valve is sutured to this patch. Postoperative complications such as regurgitation in the valve periphery or valve dehiscence sometimes occur due to weakening of the supporting tissues.

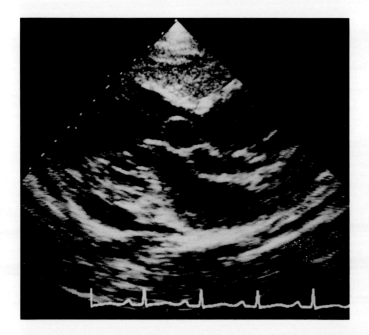

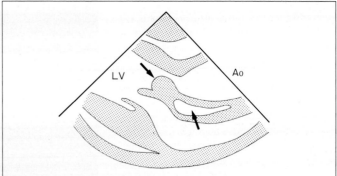

FIG. 175 Echocardiography reveals formation of a cavity extending from the aortic valvular annulus to the left ventricular outflow tract (upper arrow). An annular abscess is present (lower arrow). There is also an accumulation of pericardial fluid. (Ao, aorta; LV, left ventricle.)

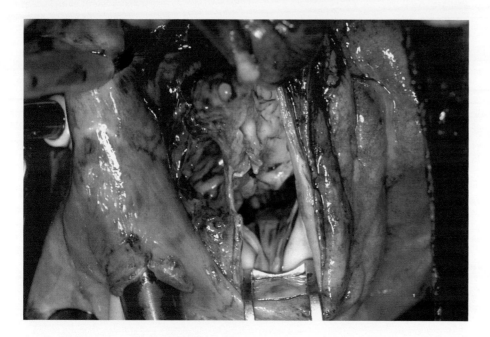

FIG. 176 Intraoperative photograph of the case discussed in Fig. 175. The annular abscess arises from the commissure between the non-coronary and left coronary cusps, extends outside the aortic wall, and forms an abscess to the wall of the left atrium. (A valve leaflet has been resected). Reconstruction of the aorta was performed in this case.

Aortic Valve Prolapse

Aortic valve prolapse does not refer to the pathophysiology of aortic valve prolapse into the left ventricle as seen in association with a variety of defects in the supporting tissues of the aortic valvular root, such as ventricular septal defect, dissecting aortic aneurysm, or traumatic lesions. Rather, aortic valve prolapse refers to myxomatous degeneration of the aortic valve itself, resulting in inadequate valvular opening and closing with subsequent development of valvular insufficiency.

Ascending aortic angiography can diagnose this disorder by detecting the presence of abnormal protrusion of the valve leaflets into the left ventricle during diastole. There may be protrusion of one or more valve leaflets. If the prolapse is severe, regurgitation develops.

Echocardiography reveals that the aortic valve deviates toward the left ventricle from its usual position of valve closure.

When Doppler techniques show deviation of the right coronary cusp into the left ventricle, there is often a regurgitant jet emitted posteriorly that strikes the anterior leaflet of the mitral valve and then reverses direction.

Originally this disorder was seen frequently in association with cystic medial necrosis of the aorta or Marfan syndrome. However, there has been a recent increase in the number of cases showing isolated involvement of the aortic valve. The etiology is unknown.

Prolapse is also seen in association with bicuspid aortic valves.

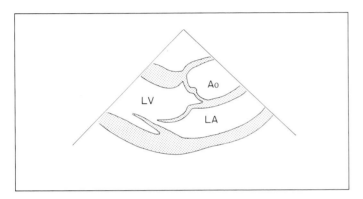

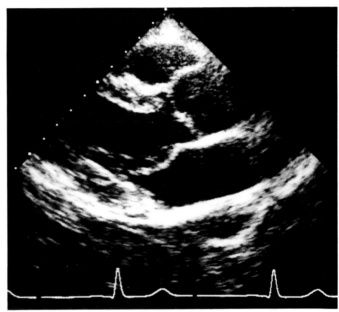

FIG. 177 Cross-sectional echocardiography along the long axis, showing deviation of the right coronary cusp into the left atrium. Even during diastole the anterior leaflet of the mitral valve does not assume an open position. This leaflet is being pushed by the regurgitant flow from the aortic valve. (Ao, aorta; LA, left atrium; LV, left ventricle.)

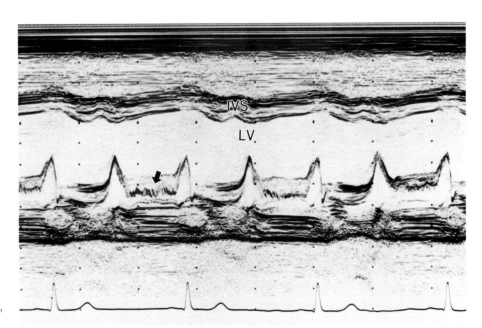

FIG. 178 M-mode echocardiography reveals fluttering of the anterior leaflet of the mitral valve due to aortic regurgitation (arrow). (IVS, interventricular septum; LV, left ventricle.)

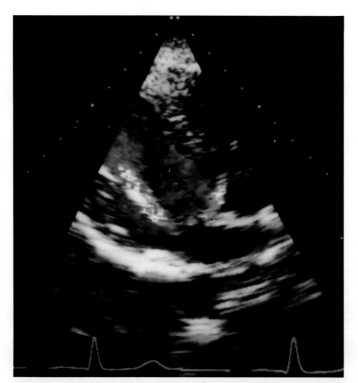

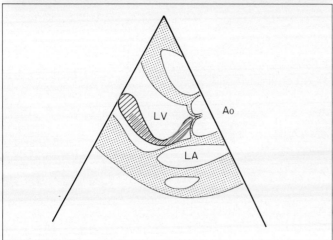

FIG. 179 Doppler imaging showing regurgitation from the aortic valve in a direction opposite to that of the prolapsing valve leaflet. The regurgitant flow strikes the anterior leaflet of the mitral valve. (Ao, aorta; LA, left atrium; LV, left ventricle.)

Aortic Insufficiency (Regurgitation) with Ventricular Septal Defect

In aortic insufficiency with ventricular septal defect, aortic angiography shows protrusion of the right coronary cusp into the right ventricular outflow tract as well as aortic regurgitation. Right ventriculography reveals a filling defect due to the right coronary cusp that protrudes into the right ventricular outflow tract. Echocardiography reveals protrusion of the right coronary cusp into the right ventricular outflow tract. Such protrusion occurs because this supraventricular crest-type ventricular septal defect is located directly below the right coronary cusp of the aortic valve.

Surgical intervention by simple closure of the ventricular septal defect is adequate if regurgitation is mild. Even in cases of moderate regurgitation, as long as there are no severe changes in the valve leaflets themselves, valvuloplasty with raising of the valve leaflets (cusp plication) has proved effective. Valve replacement is performed for cases in which regurgitation is severe.

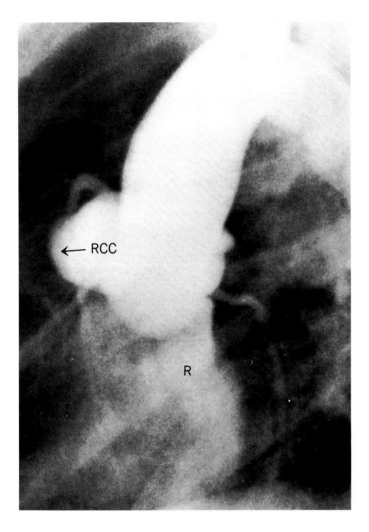

FIG. 180 Aortic angiography (lateral view) demonstrates prolapse of the right coronary cusp into the right ventricular outflow tract. Aortic regurgitation has developed between the left coronary and noncoronary cusps. (RCC, right coronary cusp; R, regurgitation.)

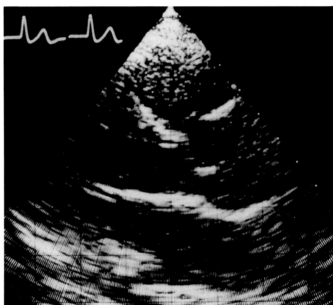

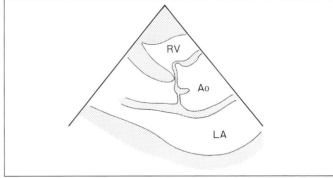

FIG. 181 Echocardiography showing aortic insufficiency with ventricular septal defect. The right coronary cusp protrudes into the left ventricular outflow tract. (Ao, aorta; LA, left atrium; RV, right ventricle.)

Annuloaortic Ectasia

Annuloaortic ectasia (AAE) is the term widely used for the pathophysiology that occurs in cases of clinically suspected aortic insufficiency in which there is sac-like enlargement of the ascending aorta and dilation of the valvular annulus, including the sinuses of Valsalva, leading to the development of aortic insufficiency. Morphologically, there is often cystic necrosis in the tunica media of the aorta. The early lesions begin in the sinuses of Valsalva. At this stage, aortic insufficiency is rare. With time the lesion reaches the origin of the aorta, and at this point aortic insufficiency appears. The dilation of the aorta usually extends to the bifurcation of the brachiocephalic trunk. The most common underlying disorder is Marfan syndrome (or an incomplete variant of Marfan syndrome). Annuloaortic ectasia is also occasionally associated with aortitis syndromes (including Takayasu arteritis), syphilis, Behçet's disease, and Ehlers-Danlos syndrome.

Aortic angiography depicts pear-shaped dilation of the aortic valve annulus and the ascending aorta superior to the annulus. If dilation of the valvular annulus is severe, aortic regurgitation is visible.

Echocardiography shows characteristic enlargement at the base of the aorta and also reveals inadequate contact of the aortic valve leaflets, with a gap present in this region.

Doppler techniques, using short-axis cross-sectional views of the regurgitant flow through the aortic valve orifice, show a triangular distribution of regurgitation toward the commissures from the center of the three aortic valve cusps. This is assumed to be from the gap that develops between the valve cusps as a result of annular dilation.

Surgical intervention is directed toward the aortic valve and the base of the aorta. An aortic root replacement is performed using a conduit attached to a prosthetic heart valve (composite graft). After grafting, there are several methods (including revised methods) for reconstruction of the openings of the right and left coronary arteries.

FIG. 182 Biopsy tissue section of the aorta, obtained during surgery of a 44-year-old man. Ten months previously, the patient developed exertional dyspnea and 7 months previously, was diagnosed with valvular disease. Beginning 5 months previously, symptoms of orthopnea and facial edema appeared. Focal loss of smooth muscle and disappearance of elastic fibers from the tunica media of the aorta are shown. There are deposits of acidic mucopolysaccharides (blue) in these areas. (Alcian blue-van Gieson stain, × 350.)

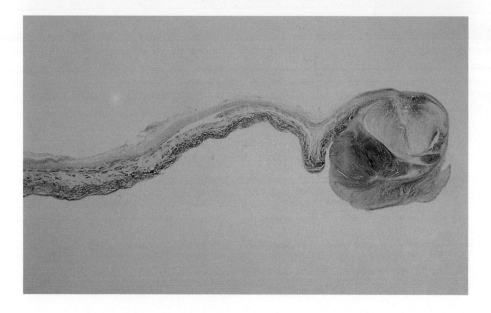

FIG. 183 Tissue section of the aortic valve from the case discussed in Fig. 182 shows nodular fibrotic thickening of the free end of the valve leaflet. The other areas of the leaflet are normal. (Alcian blue-van Gieson stain, × 17.5.)

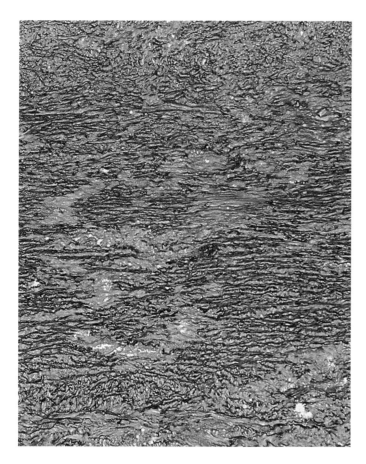

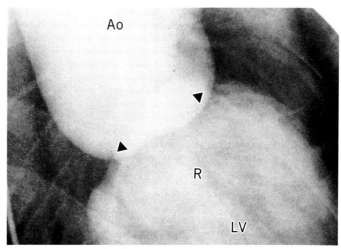

FIG. 185 Angiographic findings. Ehlers-Danlos syndrome. Aortic angiography (30-degree right oblique view) shows severe dilation of the aortic valve annulus (black arrows) and aorta. Severe regurgitation has developed. (Ao, aorta; LV, left ventricle; R, regurgitation.)

FIG. 184 Biopsy tissue section of the aorta, obtained during surgery of a 39-year-old man. Thirty-eight days previously, the patient experienced the sudden onset of severe upper abdominal pain radiating to the low back. Enlargement of the aortic valve annulus and aortic insufficiency were detected. The patient was diagnosed with a dissecting aortic aneurysm (DeBakey's classification type III). A Bentall surgical procedure was performed. Ehlers-Danlos syndrome was suspected on the basis of extensive joint hypermobility. Focal loss of smooth muscle and disappearance of elastic fibers (black stain) from the tunica media of the aorta are shown. Deposits of acidic mucopolysaccharides are present in these areas. (Elastica-van Gieson stain, × 100.)

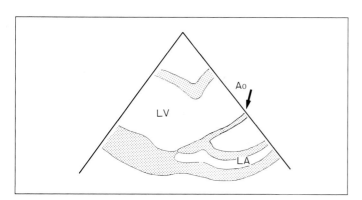

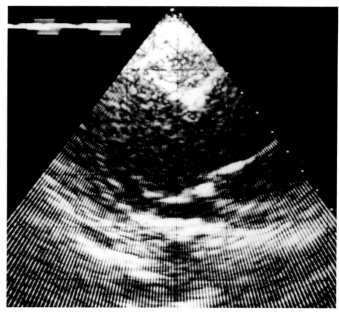

FIG. 186 Cross-sectional echocardiography along the long axis revealing marked enlargement of the aorta just superior to the aortic valve annulus. An intimal flap within the aorta due to aortic dissection (arrow) is seen. There is also left ventricular dilation as a result of aortic insufficiency. (Ao, aorta; LA, left atrium; LV, left ventricle.)

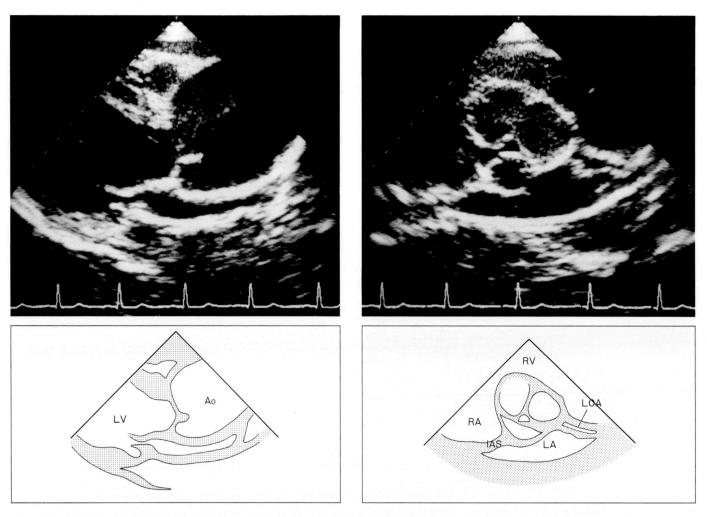

FIG. 187 (Left) Cross-sectional echocardiography along the long axis showing marked enlargement of the aorta with a peculiar configuration and dilation of the valvular annulus. (Right) Cross-sectional echocardiography along the short axis shows the development of a gap at the contact surface of the three cusps due to dilation of the annulus, resulting in regurgitant flow from this area. (Ao, aorta; IAS, interatrial septum; LA, left atrium; LCA, left coronary artery; LV, left ventricle; RA, right atrium; RV, right ventricle.)

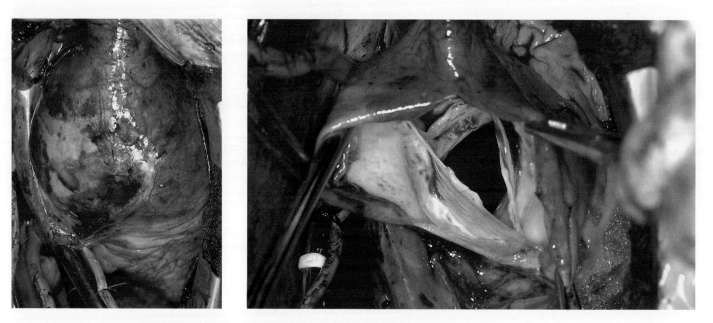

FIG. 188 Intraoperative photographs. (Left) Marked enlargement at the base of the aorta with resulting pressure on the superior vena cava and heart. (Right) Dissection of the dilated region. A triangular gap has formed between the valve cusps as a result of annular enlargement.

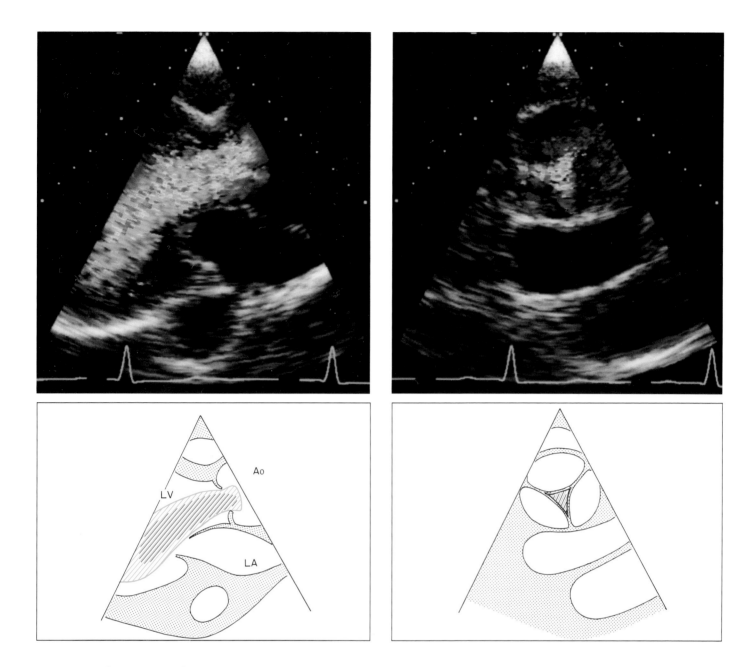

FIG. 189 Doppler imaging. (Left) A cross-sectional view along the long axis of the left
ventricle during diastole shows enlargement of the aorta. A wide regurgitant jet is
recorded from the aortic valve orifice to the left ventricle. (Right) The cross-sectional
view through the short axis of the aortic valve orifice has recorded a triangular regurgitant jet in the aortic valve orifice that is centered in the central part of the contact area
of the three cusps. This is attributed to regurgitation resulting from annular dilation.
(Ao, aorta; LA, left atrium; LV, left ventricle.)

Aortitis Syndrome

Takayasu Arteritis

In aortitis there may be extensive dilation of the ascending aorta, enlargement of the valvular annulus, and regurgitation. Although diagnostic angiography reveals extensive dilation, irregularities of the vascular walls, and severe aortic regurgitation, there may be no clear signs of enlarged valvular annulus. The characteristic findings seen in annuloaortic ectasia (AAE) are absent in this condition.

Echocardiography more commonly reveals lesions consistent with dilation than those consistent with stenosis. There is dilation of the aorta and aortic valve annulus, and the aortic valve sometimes shows mild thickening.

Surgical intervention involves valve replacement. The annular tissue is relatively rigid; it is rare for regurgitation in the periphery of the prosthetic valve (paravalvular leak) or dehiscence of the prosthetic valve (valve detachment) to develop following valve replacement. In cases in which there is marked dilation of the ascending aorta, surgical replacement of the aorta is also performed.

Pathologic and morphologic findings include (1) obstructive lesions from stenosis due to intimal thickening at the divergence of arteries from the aortic arch, (2) histologic findings of inflammation with giant cell infiltration into the tunica media, (3) intimal thickening of the nutrient blood vessels, (4) thickening in the aortic wall (mainly the tunica externa), (5) sclerosis of the aortic wall in later stages, and (6) organization of thrombi on the aortic wall.

This disorder often occurs in relatively young women.

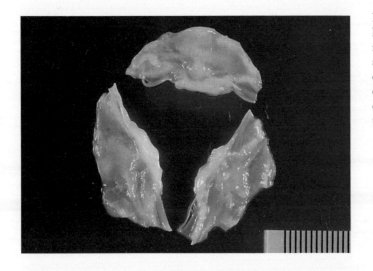

FIG. 190 Resected aortic valve of a 28-year-old woman. At age 22, she had a slight fever and developed back pain; aortitis syndrome was diagnosed. Two years previously, the patient experienced the onset of generalized fatigue, and aortic insufficiency was diagnosed. Six months previously, the patient began experiencing exertional chest pain. Elongation of the valve leaflets is seen. The free margins show "rolling" and thickening. Biopsy of the aorta, performed simultaneously, showed aortitis in the scarring stage.

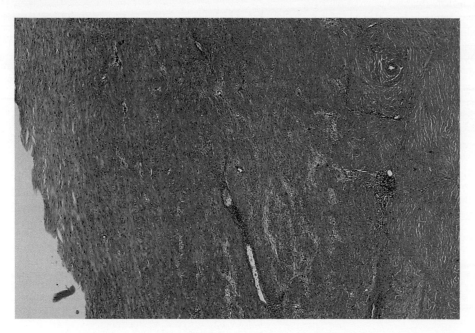

FIG. 191 Biopsy tissue section obtained during aortic surgery of a 61-year-old woman. At approximately age 51, she developed painful erythema nodosum on the left leg. At age 56, the patient experienced the onset of palpitations and dyspnea, and a diagnosis of aortic insufficiency was made. At age 58, she developed paroxysmal nocturnal dyspnea and orthopnea. Four months previously, she developed hypothyroidism with positive thyroid microsomal antibody. Aortic valve replacement was performed. Marked fibrotic thickening of the tunica intima is seen. The tunica media shows rupture and loss of the elastic fibers, an increase in collagen fibers, proliferation of the microvasculature, and lymphocytic infiltration. Marked fibrotic thickening of the tunica externa is visible, and the small vessels of the vasa vasorum show marked fibrotic thickening of the tunica intima. There is prominent lymphocytic infiltration in the periphery of the small vessels. (HE stain, × 35.)

FIG. 192 View of the left ventricular outflow tract of a 47-year-old woman after dissection of the heart along the axis of blood flow (cardiac weight 410 g). At approximately age 37, the patient experienced unexplained weight loss, and hypertension was detected. At age 44, she developed intermittent claudication, followed 1 year before death by the onset of orthopnea. Nine days before death, surgery was performed to provide a bypass and anastomosis between the descending and abdominal aorta. Although the postoperative course was initially satisfactory, hemorrhage developed from the anastomosis of the artificial vessel and the patient died. Dilation of the left ventricular cavity and endocardial thickening are shown. Tissue sections of the aorta showed probable aortitis in the scarring stage.

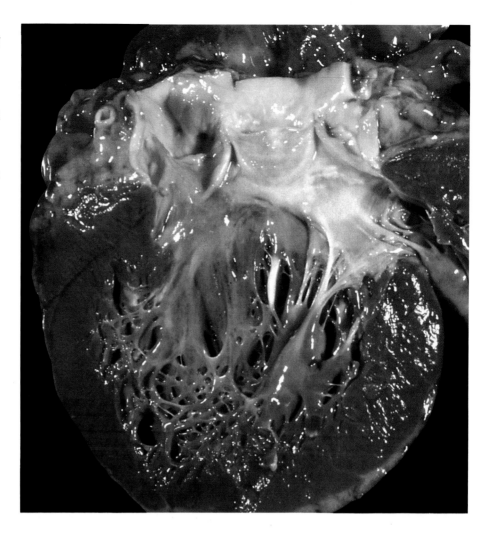

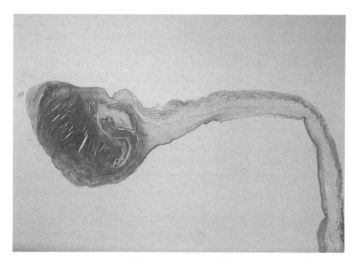

FIG. 193 Tissue section of the aortic valve of the case discussed in Fig. 191. The free margin of the valve leaflet shows nodular fibrotic thickening. The other areas of the leaflet are generally normal. (HE stain, × 13.)

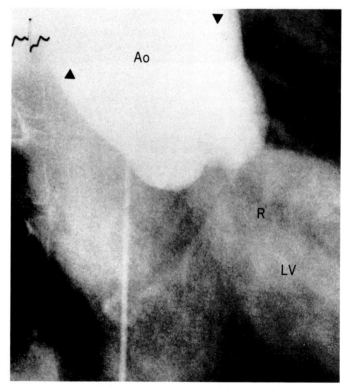

FIG. 194 Angiographic findings. Although there is no enlargement of the aortic valve annulus, regurgitation has developed due to a lesion of the valve leaflets. The aorta shows marked dilation (black arrows) above the sinus. (Ao, aorta; LV, left ventricle; R, regurgitation.)

Behçet's disease

There have been rare reports of the occurrence of aortic insufficiency in association with Behçet's disease. Lesions involving the mitral and tricuspid valves have also been reported. The male/female incidence of this condition is 2:1, with patients in their 40s most commonly affected.

Reports indicate that the etiology of aortic insufficiency in Behçet's disease is most often secondary to lesions involving the sinuses of Valsalva or the aorta, or both. However, there are also cases in which there is a primary lesion involving the aortic valve. Gross examination of the valve reveals changes varying with the particular case. These changes may be limited to mild thickening or may include degeneration and sclerosis, scar formation, perforation of the valve cusps, or valvular prolapse.

Histologic findings range in severity from limited inflammation to acute endocarditis.

There are no characteristic findings on angiography.

Echocardiography reveals mild dilation of the aorta and thickening of the aortic valve.

Although surgical valve replacement is indicated in Behçet's disease, dehiscence of the prosthetic valve often follows aortic valve replacement. Special technical procedures are required at surgery, but the most important factor in successful outcome is the use of postoperative anti-inflammatory therapy. Occasional aneurysm formation is seen near the sinuses of Valsalva, and replacement of the aortic root is also performed.

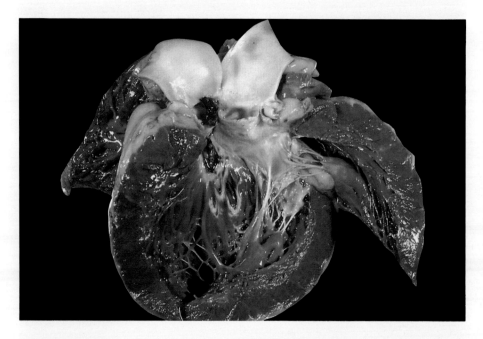

FIG. 195 View of the left ventricular inflow tract of a 49-year-old woman after dissection of the anterior wall of the left ventricle (cardiac weight 540 g). The patient developed arthralgia with swelling of the knees and feet at age 42, and ulcerations of the external genitalia at age 43. Exertional dyspnea then developed at age 48, and aortic insufficiency was diagnosed. Five months before death, Behçet's disease was also diagnosed, and steroid therapy was initiated. One week before death, the patient began to experience flu-like symptoms, and 2 days before death she had a massive bleed into the right cerebral hemisphere. Fibrotic thickening of the aortic valve cusps and the presence of large thrombotic vegetations on the right coronary cusp (infectious endocarditis) are seen. There is visible left ventricular dilation and a regurgitant jet lesion in the endocardium just below the aortic valve.

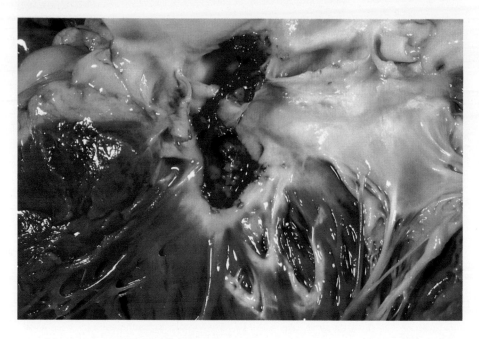

FIG. 196 Close-up view of the aortic valve from the case discussed in Fig. 195, showing fibrotic thickening of the aortic valve cusps and a large thrombotic vegetation on the right coronary cusp. Microscopic examination revealed prominent neutrophilic infiltration (infectious endocarditis). A regurgitant jet lesion was noted just below the aortic valve.

Calcific Aortic Stenosis

Echocardiography in cases of calcific aortic stenosis reveals clinical findings of thickening, decreased mobility, enhanced luminance, and calcification of the aortic valve. The commissures are not fused. Stenosis produces left ventricular wall hypertrophy and narrowing of the left ventricular cavity.

When depicting valvular calcification, cineangiography shows virtually no movement of the valve leaflets and only slight opening of the valve orifice.

The following points should be considered in distinguishing morphologically pure calcific (senile) aortic stenosis from rheumatic aortic stenosis. First, in rheumatic aortic stenosis, there is fusion of the commissures and secondary calcification that often involves the lateral one-third of the free valve margins. Commonly, concomitant rheumatic lesions of the mitral valve are visible. Second, calcific aortic stenosis is significantly more frequent in elderly men; the calcification begins and is concentrated in the bases of the sinuses of Valsalva. Third, in calcific (senile) stenosis the fibrous layer on the aortic side of the valvular velum is the primary site where calcification develops. By contrast, calcification in rheumatic related stenosis involves primarily the spongy and ventricular layers in the ventricular aspect of the valve. Finally, atheromas (xanthomatous lesions) are visible, with occasional sclerosis.

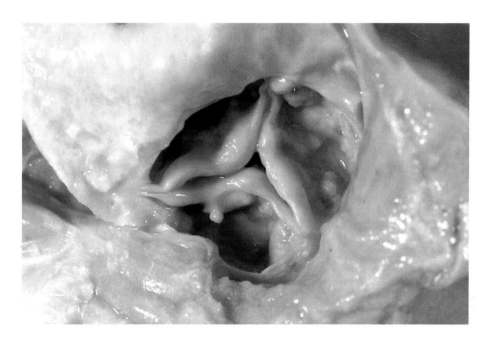

FIG. 197 View of the aortic valve from the aortic side (cardiac weight 450 g) of a 74-year-old woman. Treatment for hypertension was initiated at age 64. Three years before death, the patient developed symptoms of exertional angina and 7 months before death, was diagnosed with aortic insufficiency. Although she received medical therapy, she eventually died due to progressive worsening of heart failure. Fibrotic thickening of the valve cusps and multiple calcified deposits within the aortic (Valsalva) sinuses are shown. There is no fusion of the commissures. The aorta shows signs of atherosclerosis.

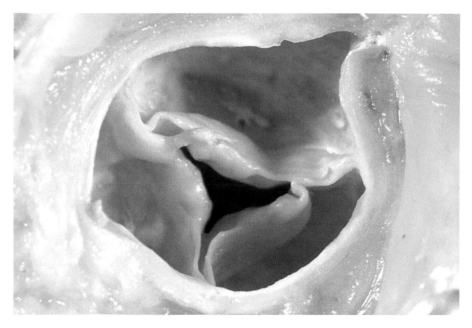

FIG. 198 View of the aortic valve from the aortic side of an 87-year-old woman. The patient was diagnosed with hypertension 10 years before death. She died as a result of a cerebellar hemorrhage. Although echocardiography revealed sclerotic findings of the aortic valve, there were no abnormalities of the mitral valve.

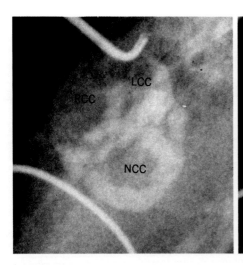 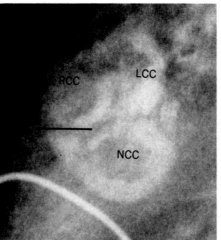

FIG. 199 Aortic angiography, 60-degree left anterior oblique view. (Left) During diastole, severe calcification of the aortic valve cusps and annulus is seen. (Right) During systole, a narrow slit-like opening (O) between the right coronary and noncoronary cusps is seen. There is fusion, with no opening, between the right coronary and left coronary cusps and between the left coronary and noncoronary cusps. (LCC, left coronary cusp; NCC, noncoronary cusp; RCC, right coronary cusp.)

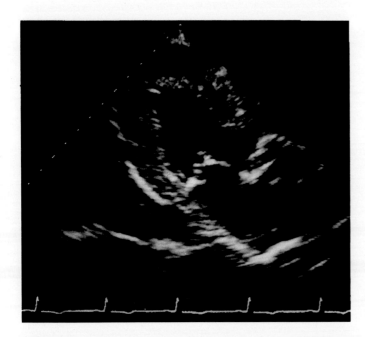

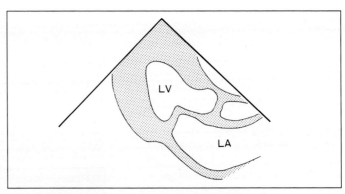

FIG. 200 Cross-sectional echocardiography along the long axis from the cardiac apex shows thickening of the aortic valve. Hypertrophy of the left ventricular wall and interventricular septum is present. (LA, left atrium; LV, left ventricle.)

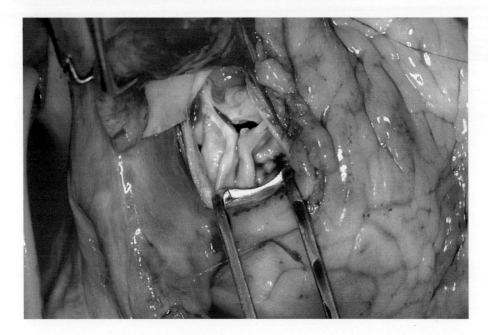

FIG. 201 Intraoperative photograph showing thickening of the valve cusps but no fusion of the commissures. There is prominent sclerosis of the three valve cusps with marked restriction of valve opening.

Familial Hypercholesterolemia

Xanthomatous deposits and thickening of the aortic valve, although rare, are seen in familial hypercholesterolemias. These changes can lead to aortic valvular dysfunction. Although xanthomatous deposits can similarly affect the mitral valve, they rarely involve the tricuspid and pulmonary valves. In cases of familial hypercholesterolemia, atherosclerotic lesions characteristically appear at the origin of the aorta and the aortic arch. Stenotic lesions develop not only on the aortic valve but also at the openings of the coronary arteries.

Aortic angiography reveals irregularities involving the surface of the aortic valve cusps, the proximal ascending aorta, the opening of the coronary arteries, and the aortic arch.

Echocardiography shows thickening of the aortic valve and the wall of the aorta. Occasionally, thickening of the mitral valve is also seen.

In this condition there is generally coexistent supravalvular stenosis and stenosis of the openings of the coronary arteries. Surgical intervention requires aortic root replacement using a conduit attached to a prosthetic heart valve, along with reconstruction of the coronary arteries.

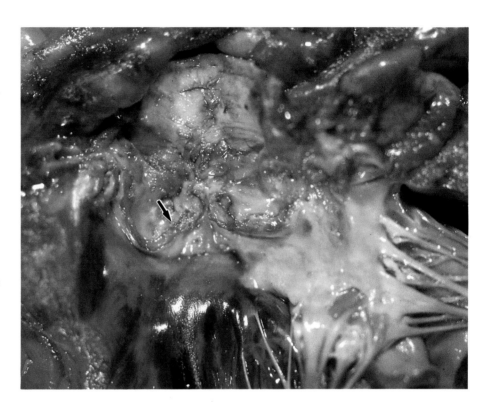

FIG. 202 View of the aortic valve following dissection of the left ventricular outflow tract (cardiac weight 560 g) of a 21-year-old woman. At age 3, xanthomas appeared on both Achilles tendons, and at age 8, she developed xanthomas on both elbows and both knees. At age 12, hypertension and a heart murmur were detected. At age 13, the patient experienced the onset of left anterior chest discomfort after walking for approximately 15 minutes. One year before death, she was diagnosed with type IIa familial hyperlipoproteinemia (homozygous), along with impairment of intracellular low density lipoprotein (LDL) uptake. Aortic stenosis was also present. Two days before death, the patient underwent an aortic-coronary artery bypass and Bentall procedure and subsequently died from low cardiac output syndrome. Deformation of the aortic valve (arrow) due to pressure on the wall from surgery is shown. There are prominent xanthomatous deposits on the mitral valve.

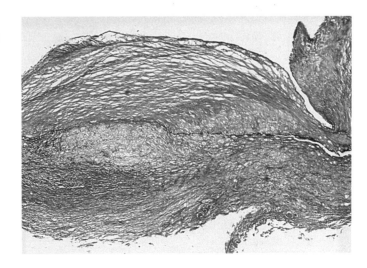

FIG. 203 Tissue section of the aortic valve of the case discussed in Fig. 202 (Fig. 202, arrow). The central portion of the valve shows xanthoma formation. (HE stain, × 50.)

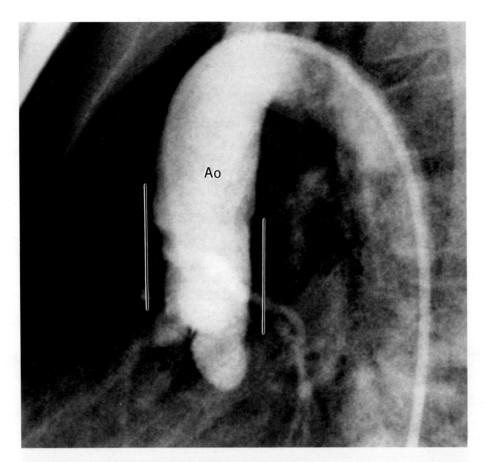

FIG. 204 Aortic angiography (lateral view) depicting irregular sclerotic lesions (side lines) of the aortic wall due to atherosclerosis with fatty deposits. (Ao, ascending aorta.)

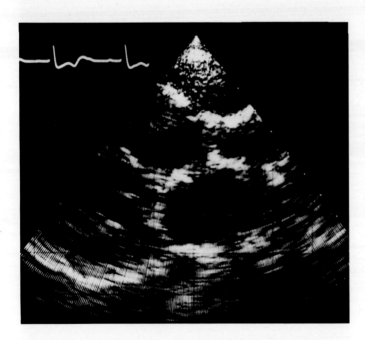

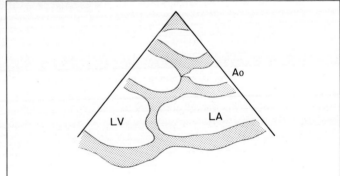

FIG. 205 Cross-sectional echocardiography along the long axis showing thickening of the aortic valve, the mitral valve, and the wall of the aorta. (Ao, aorta; LA, left atrium; LV, left ventricle.)

Nonbacterial Thrombotic Endocarditis

Nonbacterial thrombotic endocarditis occurs most frequently in the mitral valve, followed by the aortic and tricuspid valves.

There are basically no marked differences in clinical presentation between those cases affecting the mitral valve and those affecting the other valves. Nonbacterial thrombotic endocarditis of the aortic valve frequently develops near the Arantius' nodules. See Chapter 2 for further details.

FIG. 206 View of the aortic valve (cardiac weight 470 g) of a 63-year-old man diagnosed 2 years previously with hypertension. Nine days before death, the patient developed sudden left hemiplegia, was hospitalized, and died of cerebral edema. Autopsy revealed carcinoma of the prostate, nonbacterial thrombotic endocarditis of the aortic valve, and obstruction of the cerebral arteries due to emboli. Clusters of thrombotic vegetations near the Arantius' nodules of the valvular cusps are seen.

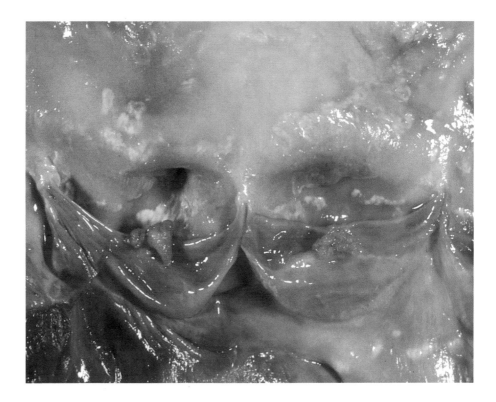

FIG. 207 View of the aortic valve (cardiac weight 490 g) of a 71-year-old man. At age 61, cardiac arrhythmia and hypertension were detected. One month before death, the patient was hospitalized with right hemiplegia; during hospitalization he developed bloody bowel movements and DIC and death ensued. Abdominal echocardiography revealed a tumor in the gallbladder. Autopsy showed carcinoma of the gallbladder (moderately differentiated adenocarcinoma). Granular thrombotic vegetations of the surface along the closed margins of the valve are seen.

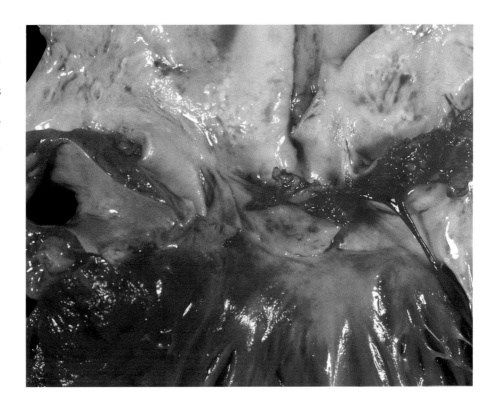

IV
Tricuspid Valvular Disease

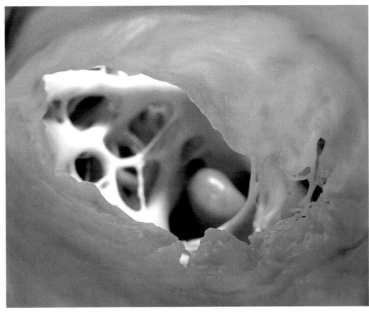

Tricuspid valve of a 19-year-old woman with primary pulmonary hypertension. There is notable thinning of the valve leaflets, marked dilation of the right ventricle, and thrombus formation in the apex.

Rheumatic Valvular Disease

Although stenosis and insufficiency are known to occur in the tricuspid valve, the other valves are more often affected by rheumatic disease, and isolated involvement of the tricuspid valve is rare.

Tricuspid stenosis develops because of rheumatic inflammatory changes in the commissures, with resulting adhesion of the valve leaflets. There is concomitant marked dilation of the right atrium with hypertrophy of the right atrial wall due to increased blood volume in the right atrium during diastole. In tricuspid insufficiency, rheumatic inflammatory changes lead to enlargement and thickening of the leaflets with a resultant loss of mobility and inadequate valve closure. Fusion of the leaflets occurs at their adjacent free margins, with closure of each commissure, and eventually the rigid valvular orifice takes on the shape of a shallow "tunnel." Regurgitation then develops at the orifice of the tricuspid valve, and cardiac output is markedly decreased.

Echocardiography shows thickening of the tricuspid valve, restriction of valve opening, and dome formation. Regurgitant lesions are more prominent than stenotic lesions.

It is rare to see severe thickening and calcification such as occur in the mitral valve. The surgical approach of valvuloplasty, using a combination of a commissurotomy and annuloplasty, is of limited applicability here. In cases involving shortening of the valve cusps (small leaflet area), valve replacement using a tissue valve is performed.

See Chapter 2 for a discussion of pathologic and morphologic findings.

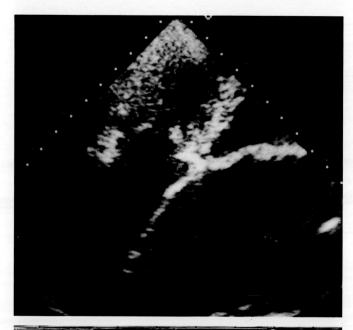

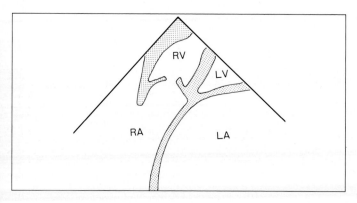

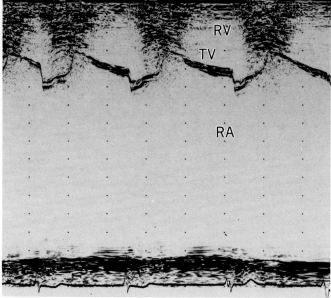

FIG. 208 (Top) Four-chamber cross-sectional echocardiography shows sclerosis and restriction of the opening of the tricuspid valve. In rheumatic valvular disease, stenotic lesions are often accompanied by regurgitation. (Bottom) M-mode echocardiography shows valve thickening. Findings of decreased mobility resemble those seen in mitral valves. (LA, left atrium; LV, left ventricle; RA, right atrium; RV, right ventricle; TV, tricuspid valve.)

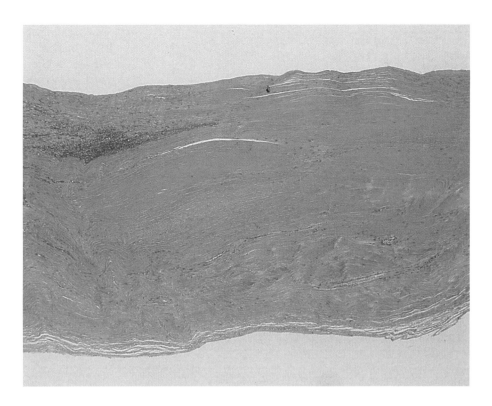

FIG. 209 Tissue section of a resected tricuspid valve of a 62-year-old woman. At age 31, the patient developed cardiomegaly, at approximately age 38, the onset of exertional dyspnea was noted, and at age 57, the aortic and mitral valves were replaced. At age 62, symptoms of valvular incompetence developed, and the patient underwent another replacement procedure. During surgery, fusion of the tricuspid valve commissures was noted. Diffuse fibrotic thickening of the valve leaflets accompanied by microvascular proliferation is shown. (HE stain, × 35.)

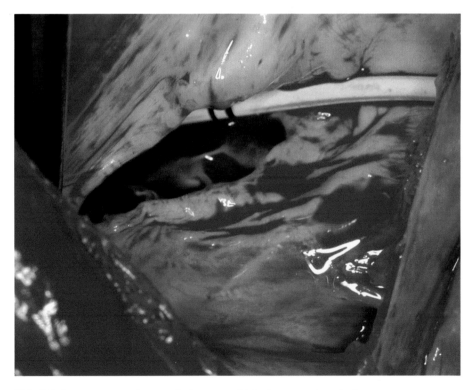

FIG. 210 Intraoperative photograph showing mild thickening and marked shortening of the valve leaflets. There is noticeable fusion of the posterior and septal leaflets.

Traumatic Insufficiency (Regurgitation)

There is a long history of documentation of etiologies in the development of traumatic valvular insufficiency, including cardiac trauma with a blunt instrument, motor vehicle accidents, and cardiac resuscitation, so it is known that injury to the supporting tissues of the tricuspid valve can lead to insufficiency.

Echocardiography reveals flopping of the valve into the right atrium in association with rupture of the chordae tendineae.

Surgical interventions, such as repair of ruptured chordae tendineae or valvuloplasty in the case of ruptured chordae tendineae with associated mitral valve prolapse, have been successful.

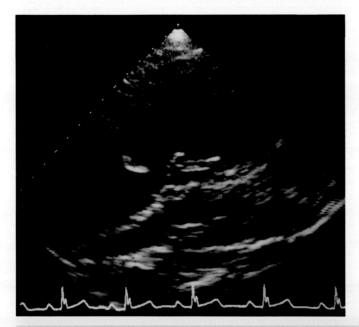

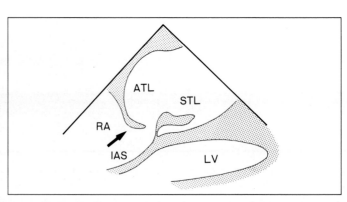

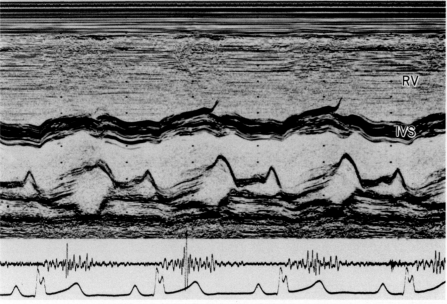

FIG. 211 Echocardiography. (Top) Inversion of the anterior leaflet of the tricuspid valve into the right atrium (arrow). Most cases of tricuspid valve prolapse show a lesser degree of prolapse than is demonstrated here, suggesting that rupture of the chordae tendineae should be considered. There is also marked dilation of the right ventricle and right atrium, and the interatrial septum is pushed from the right atrium into the left atrium. (Bottom) M-mode echocardiography shows dilation of the right ventricle and paradoxical motion of the interventricular septum. Right ventricular volume overload resulting from tricuspid valve insufficiency is indicated. (ATL, anterior leaflet of the tricuspid valve; IAS, interatrial septum; IVS, interventricular septum; LV, left ventricle; RA, right atrium; RV, right ventricle; STL, septal leaflet of the tricuspid valve.)

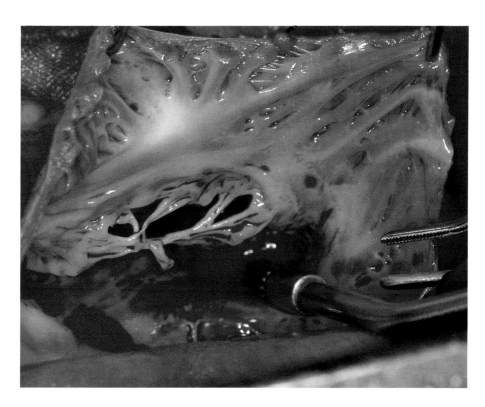

FIG. 212 Intraoperative photograph showing rupture of the chordae tendineae of the anterior and posterior leaflets. Surgical repair was performed by suturing and annuloplasty after triangular resection of the prolapsed portion of the valve.

Secondary Tricuspid Insufficiency (Regurgitation)

Secondary tricuspid insufficiency is most frequently associated with pathophysiology involving right ventricular dilation in cases of pulmonary hypertension. Secondary insufficiency is also known to occur as a complication of conditions, including infective endocarditis, myocardial infarction, carcinoid syndrome, and atrial septal defects.

In this condition, right ventriculography reveals regurgitation into the right atrium. Accurate evaluation by angiography of valvular ring enlargement and the area of regurgitation is essential. Echocardiography shows insufficient closure of the valve due to enlargement of the tricuspid valvular ring.

Doppler techniques are used to evaluate the region from the tricuspid valve orifice to within the right atrium using parasternal four-chamber cross-sectional views and cross-sectional views of the inflow tract of the right ventricle, and to record the signal due to regurgitation into the right atrium from the tricuspid valve orifice during systole. The area of regurgitation is then measured from the largest cross-section recording. Using these indicators, regurgitation in the left side of the heart can similarly be classified into four stages (degrees) of regurgitation. Continuous-wave Doppler methods are also used to measure the maximum flow velocity or regurgitation. Right ventricular systolic pressure can be measured using a simplified form of Bernoulli's method.

Although several forms of surgical intervention are available, annuloplasty is selected in almost all cases. Where there is exceptionally severe right-sided heart failure, valve replacement surgery is occasionally performed to obtain full valvular function.

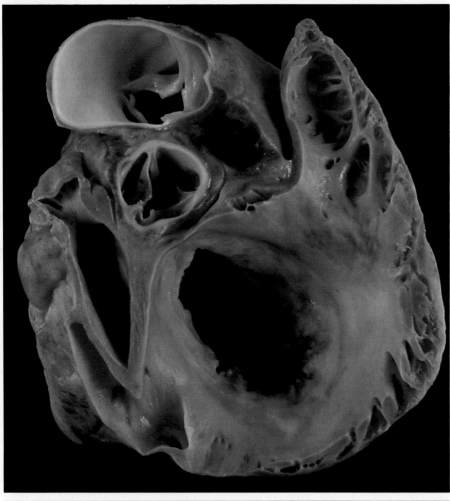

FIG. 213 View from above the heart of a 19-year-old woman after dissection of the left and right atria (cardiac weight 330 g). At age 11, the patient developed exertional dyspnea and at age 12, was diagnosed with primary pulmonary hypertension. Death occurred 3 days after a rapid overall worsening of condition. The right atrium is markedly dilated in comparison to the left atrium. There is prominent enlargement of the tricuspid valve ring, and the pulmonary artery is also enlarged in comparison to the aorta.

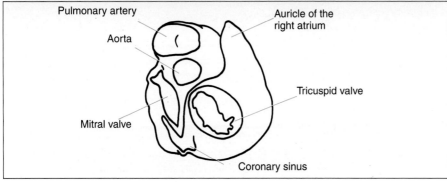

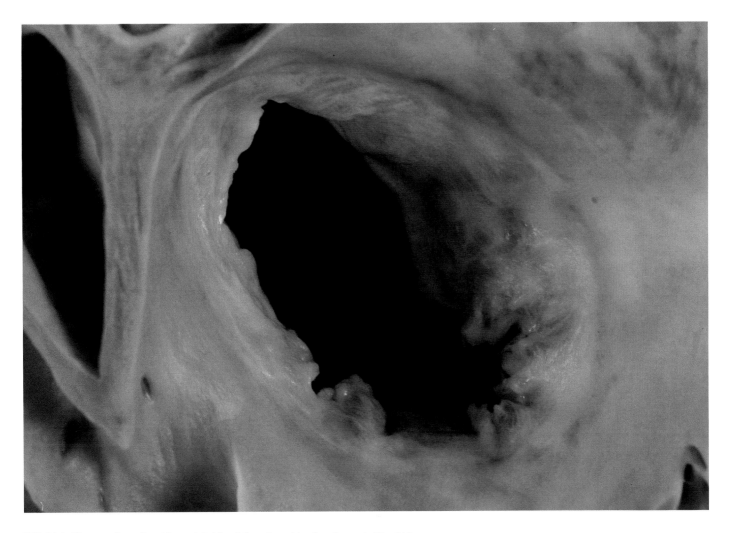

FIG. 214 Close-up from the right atrial side of the tricuspid valve shown in Fig. 213. The tricuspid valve ring is enlarged, with involvement of the margin of the valve.

FIG. 215 Imaging from left ventriculography. A regurgitant jet is visible, emitted upward from the tricuspid valve into the posterior wall of the right atrium. (PA, pulmonary artery; rj, regurgitant jet; RV, right ventricle.)

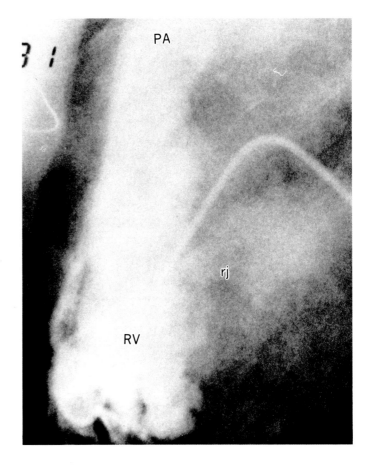

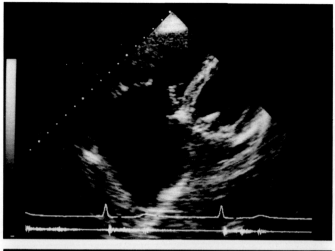

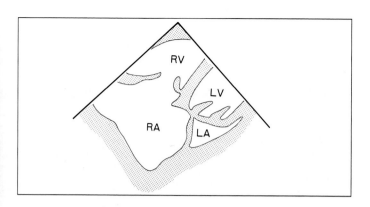

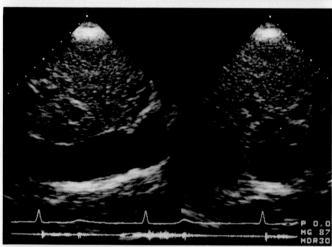

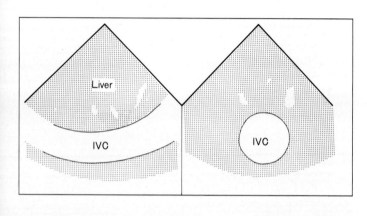

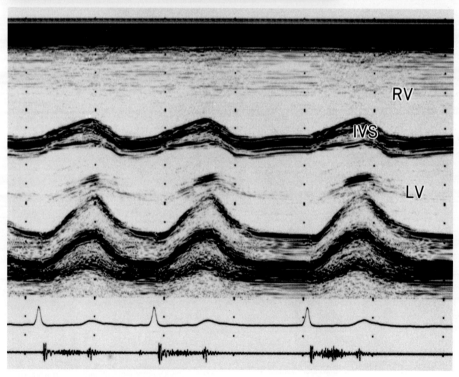

FIG. 216 Echocardiography. Tricuspid valvular insufficiency was noted after replacement of the aortic and mitral valves. (Top) Four-chamber cross-sectional echocardiography shows an opening between the anterior and septal leaflets of the tricuspid valve that is present even during systole. The interatrial septum is pushed into the side of the left atrium by the dilated right atrium. (Middle) Enlargement of the inferior vena cava. (Bottom) M-mode echocardiography indicates paradoxical motion of the dilated right ventricle and the interventricular septum. (IVC, inferior vena cava; IVS, interventricular septum; LA, left atrium; LV, left ventricle; RA, right atrium; RV, right ventricle.)

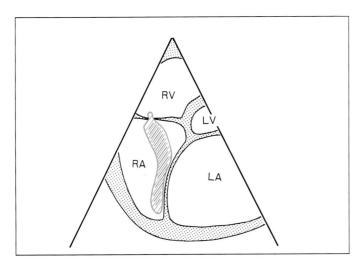

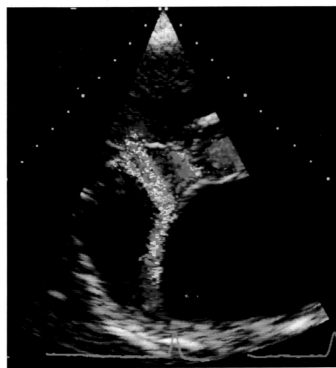

FIG. 217 Doppler imaging. A parasternal four-chamber cross-sectional view during systole. A regurgitant jet is recorded from the center of the tricuspid valve orifice into the right atrium. The jet is striking the interatrial septum, which is projecting into the right ventricle because of left atrial enlargement. The direction of the regurgitation is changed (secondary tricuspid insufficiency with regurgitation from the center of the valvular orifice). Using the width of the regurgitant jet as an indicator, the degree of regurgitation can be evaluated on a four-stage scale. (LA, left atrium; LV, left ventricle; RA, right atrium; RV, right ventricle.)

Infectious Endocarditis

Please refer to Chapter 2 for clinical information and pathologic and morphologic findings.

Valve replacement is performed during the active phase of an infection. In the healing phase such replacement is rarely conducted as a separate surgical procedure, although valvuloplasty is commonly performed.

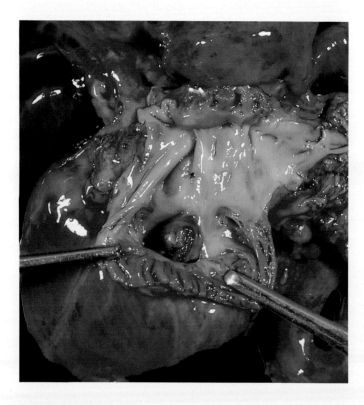

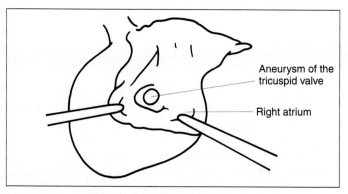

FIG. 218 View of the tricuspid valve after dissection of the right atrium. The patient was a 4-month-old infant girl. After birth, a cardiac murmur and tachypnea were detected, and aortic coarctation was diagnosed. On day 12 after birth, the patient underwent surgical repair of the aorta. On day 67, a patch closure procedure was performed for a ventricular septal defect. Postoperative mediastinitis then developed, requiring management with mechanical ventilation. Thirty-seven days before death, vegetations were noted near the tricuspid valve. Twenty-six days before death, the patient developed acute hepatitis; death resulted from hepatic failure. Formation of a large aneurysm in the tricuspid valve is shown.

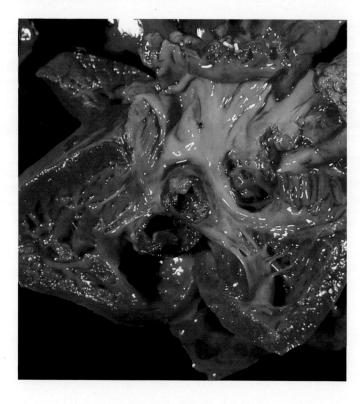

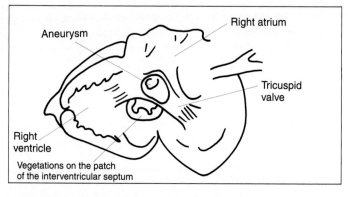

FIG. 219 View of the tricuspid valve after dissection of the posterior wall of the right ventricle of the case discussed in Fig. 218. A large aneurysm is visible, with dome-like protrusion into the anterior leaflet of the tricuspid valve.

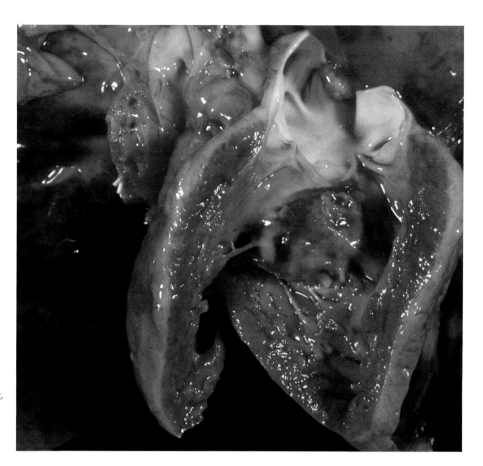

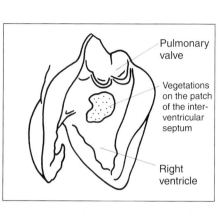

Pulmonary valve

Vegetations on the patch of the interventricular septum

Right ventricle

FIG. 220 View after dissection of the right ventricular outflow tract of the case discussed in Fig. 218. A large thrombotic vegetation can be seen protruding into the right ventricular outflow tract near the region of the membranous part of the interventricular septum. This area corresponds to the area of patch closure of the ventricular septal defect. The partially displaced patch is visible within the vegetation.

FIG. 221 Intraoperative photograph. A large vegetation has formed on the septal leaflet; the infection is in its active stage. In this case, a valve replacement was performed after resection of the valve leaflet.

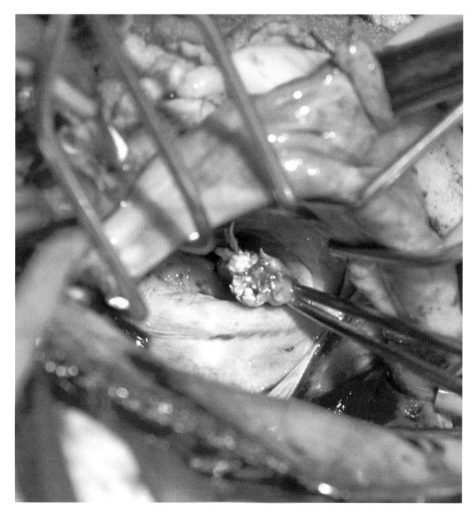

Miscellaneous

The case discussed in this section as "miscellaneous" is a case identified as tricuspid valvular regurgitation on the basis of the presence of marked fatty infiltration in the right and left ventricles noted on dissected specimens after surgical valve replacement. Although a variety of etiologies can lead to regurgitation, cases such as this, in which regurgitation develops as a result of myocardial lesions with fatty infiltration, are rare.

Illustrations are from the case of a 66-year-old woman who had a 30-year history of heart failure.

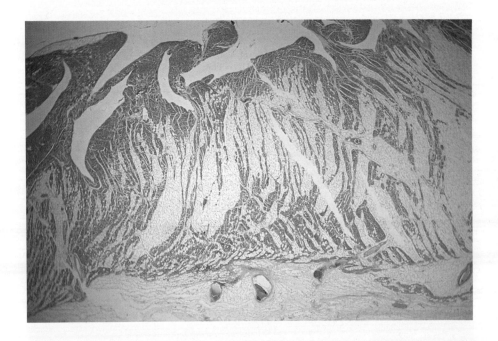

FIG. 222 Tissue section of the anterior wall of the right ventricle of a 66-year-old woman. At approximately age 36, the patient developed facial and lower extremity edema as well as symptoms of exertional dyspnea. At age 47, she was diagnosed with tricuspid valvular insufficiency and at age 57, experienced recurring symptoms of heart failure. Four days before death, both the tricuspid and mitral valves were replaced, after which the patient developed symptoms of low cardiac output and subsequently died. The walls of the right ventricle show marked fatty infiltration. The myocardial bundles have a reed-like appearance. There is little fatty infiltration into the trabeculae. (HE stain.)

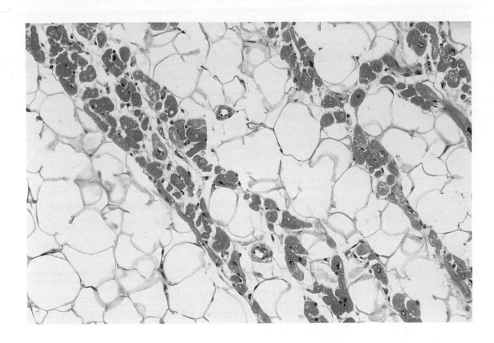

FIG. 223 Tissue section from the anterior wall of the right ventricle of the case discussed in Fig. 222. Marked fatty infiltration can be seen. (HE stain, × 175.)

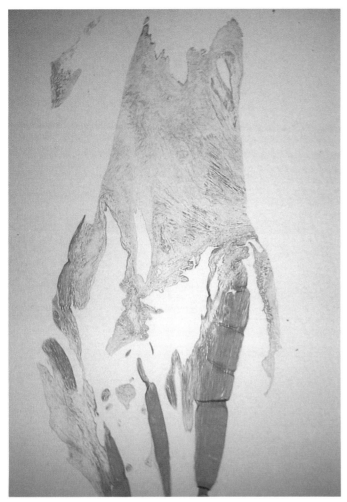

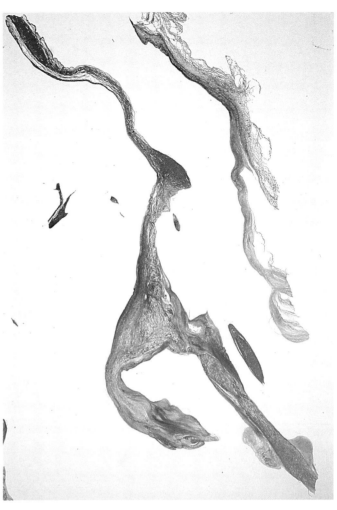

FIG. 224 Tissue section from the mitral valve of the case discussed in Fig. 222. Prominent myxomatous changes of the leaflets are visible, and the chordae tendineae are fibrotic.

FIG. 225 Tissue section of the mitral valve from the case discussed in Fig. 222. Prominent myxomatous changes of the leaflets are visible, and the chordae tendineae are fibrotic. (Elastica-van Gieson stain.)

FIG. 226 Intraoperative photograph of the case discussed in Fig. 222.

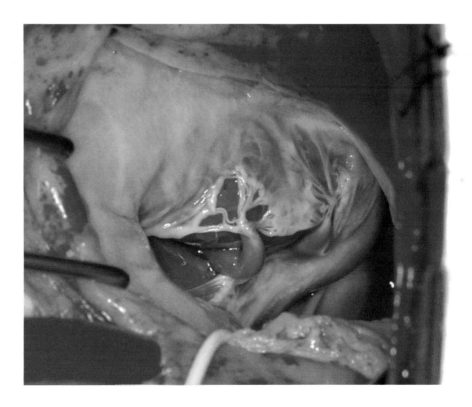

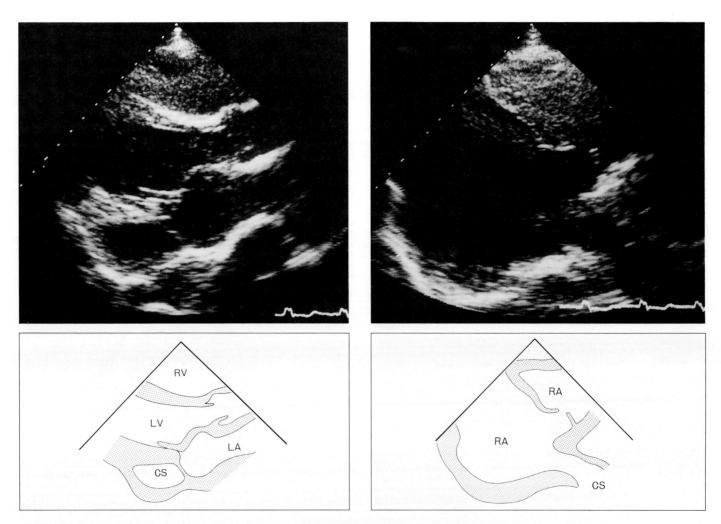

FIG. 227 Echocardiogram of the case discussed in Fig. 222. (Left) Displacement of the anterior leaflet of the mitral valve into the left atrium, with mitral valve prolapse. There is notable enlargement of the coronary sinus due to a remnant of the left side of the superior vena cava. (Right) A gap between the anterior and septal leaflets of the tricuspid valve and marked enlargement of the right atrium are present. (CS, coronary sinus; LA, left atrium; LV, left ventricle; RA, right atrium; RV, right ventricle.)

V
Pulmonary Valvular Disease

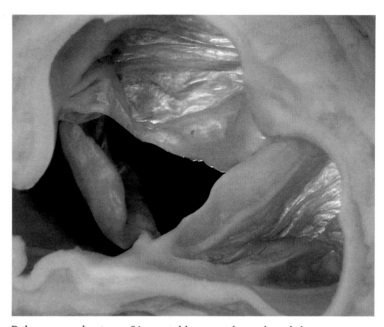

Pulmonary valve in an 81-year-old man with combined rheumatic valvular disease. There is elongation and thinning of the valve leaflets and involvement of the free margins of the valve.

The incidence of acquired pulmonary valvular disease is low in comparison to other valve disease, and stenotic changes in the pulmonary valve itself are rare. However, the presence of stenosis in either the supravalvular or subvalvular region leads to pathophysiologic findings that are hemodynamically similar to valvular stenosis.

Diseases such as rheumatic fever, infective endocarditis, and carcinoid syndrome can produce stenosis and insufficiency of the pulmonary valve itself. In addition, the location of the pulmonary valve makes it prone to the effects of intrathoracic mediastinal tumors and malignant lesions involving the right ventricular outflow tract.

Congenital Pulmonary Stenosis

Right ventriculography reveals dome formation in the pulmonary valve, emission of a narrow jet of blood from the center of this area, and poststenotic ectasia of the pulmonary trunk. The right ventricular outflow tract generally shows severe muscular hypertrophy and infundibular stenosis.

Echocardiography shows dome formation due to fusion of the pulmonary valve accompanied by hypertrophy of the right ventricular wall.

Surgical intervention in the form of commissurotomy offers a good prognosis in most cases, although there may be some degree of residual stenosis and insufficiency. It is important that the procedure be extended as far as the valvular ring. There are also cases in which dilation of the supravalvular area of the pulmonary artery or subvalvular area of the infundibulum (or both) is required.

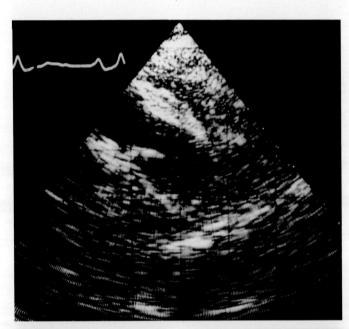
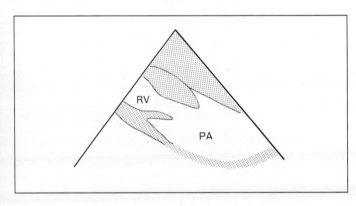
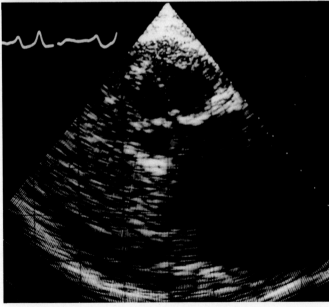
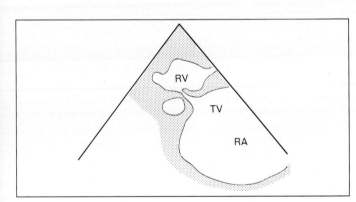

FIG. 228 Echocardiography of pulmonary stenosis. (Top) Thickening of the pulmonary valve and restricted valve opening can be observed. (Bottom) No notable lesions of the tricuspid valve are seen, but there is visible thickening of the right ventricular wall and dilation of the right atrium. (PA, pulmonary artery; RA, right atrium; RV, right ventricle; TV, tricuspid valve.)

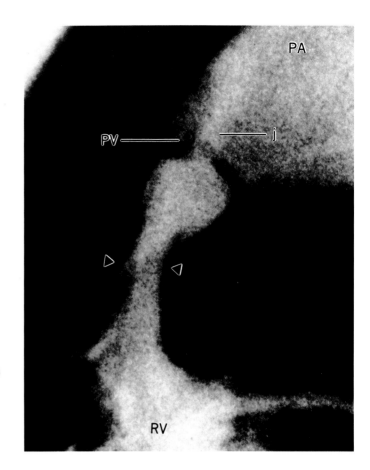

FIG. 229 Right ventriculography (lateral view) showing severe stenosis of the pulmonary valve. The jet from the center of the valve is emitted toward the upper wall of the pulmonary trunk. There is some post-stenotic ectasia of the pulmonary artery and secondary hypertrophy in the right ventricular infundibulum (black triangle). (j; jet; PA, pulmonary artery; PV, pulmonary valve; RV, right ventricle.)

FIG. 230 Intraoperative photograph. Observation of the pulmonary valve after dissection of the pulmonary artery reveals marked thickening of the valve leaflets and severe fusion of each commissure. In this case, commissurotomy and debridement were performed.

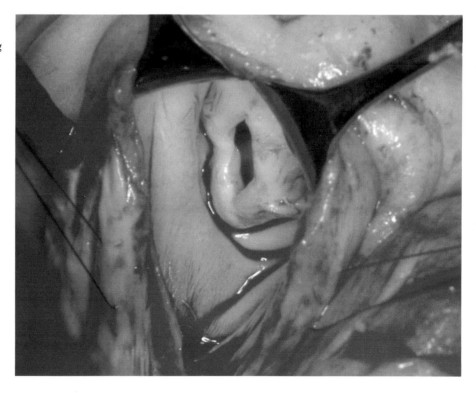

Infectious Endocarditis

Echocardiography shows vegetations on the pulmonary valve. This patient had an underlying ventricular septal defect and patent ductus arteriosus (Figs. 231 and 232). A valvuloplasty was performed with removal of the vegetations on the pulmonary valve and closure of the perforation. Valve replacement using tissue valves is done only in adults who have significant damage to the valvular tissue.

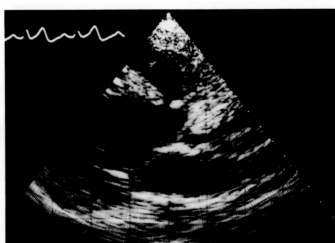

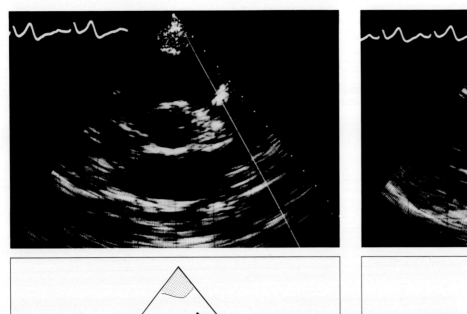

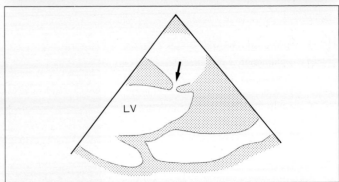

FIG. 231 Echocardiography of vegetations on the pulmonary valve and a ventricular septal defect. (Left) Cross-sectional echocardiography in the direction of the right ventricular outflow tract shows vegetations on the pulmonary valve (arrow). (Right) Cross-sectional echocardiog- raphy along the long axis reveals a type I ventricular septal defect between the aorta and the interventricular septum (arrow). (Ao, aorta; LA, left atrium; LV, left ventricle; PA, pulmonary artery; RA, right atrium; RV, right ventricle.)

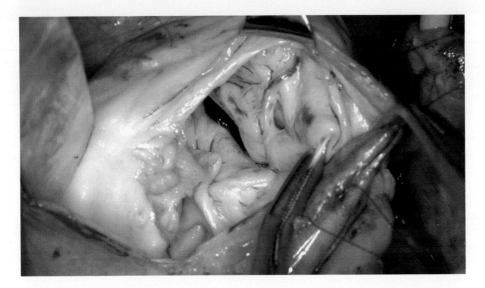

FIG. 232 Intraoperative photograph. A ventricular septal defect with a diameter of approximately 6 mm is visible below the pulmonary valve. The periphery is covered with fibrotic tissue. In this case, the ventricular septal defect was repaired by patch closure, and the pulmonary valve was replaced with a tissue valve.

Secondary Insufficiency (Regurgitation)

Doppler techniques permit evaluation of the central part of the pulmonary valve orifice by means of a cross-section along the long axis of the right ventricular outflow tract, and recording of the signal of jet-like regurgitation from the pulmonary valve orifice into the right ventricular outflow tract during diastole. By using the continuous-wave Doppler method to measure maximum flow velocity and then applying a simplified form of Bernoulli's method, end-diastolic pressure in the pulmonary artery can be estimated.

The etiology of regurgitation in this case was enlargement of the pulmonary artery at the commissural level. Plication of this region, done from outside the wall of the pulmonary artery, can be highly effective in such cases.

FIG. 233 Right anterior view of the heart. At age 11, the patient developed symptoms of exertional dyspnea and at age 12, primary pulmonary hypertension was diagnosed. The patient's general condition deteriorated suddenly 3 days before death. Marked dilation of the right atrium and right ventricle is shown.

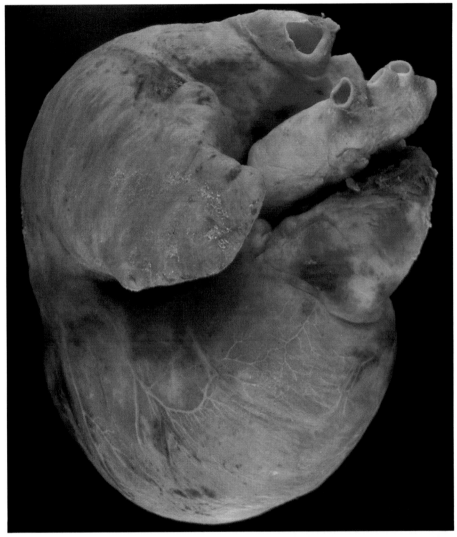

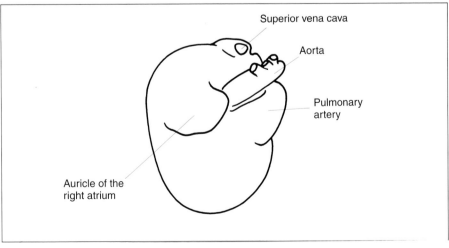

Superior vena cava

Aorta

Pulmonary artery

Auricle of the right atrium

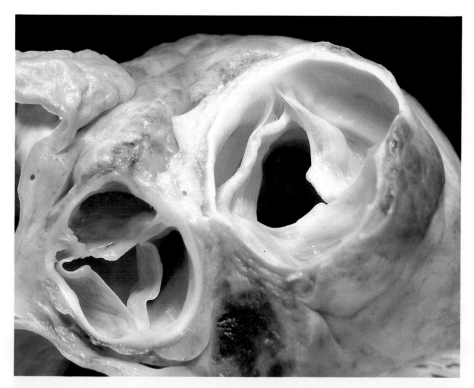

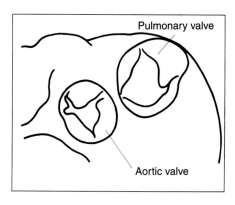

FIG. 234 View from the arterial side of the aortic and pulmonary valves of the case discussed in Fig. 233. The pulmonary artery is markedly dilated in comparison to the aorta. The leaflets of the pulmonary valve are elongated, and there is involvement of the valve margin with thickening.

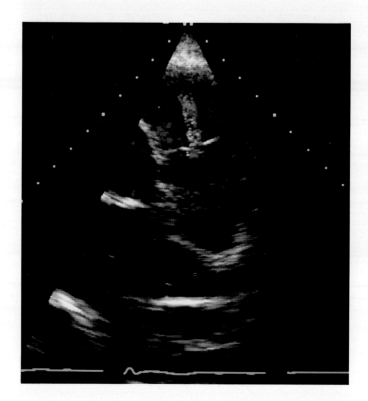

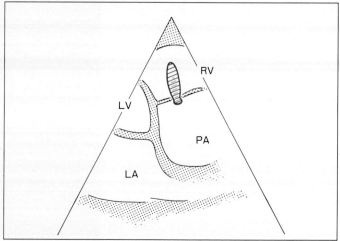

FIG. 235 Doppler imaging. A horizontal cross-section from the right ventricular outflow tract to the pulmonary artery. A narrow jet-like regurgitant signal is recorded from the center of the pulmonary valve orifice to the right ventricular outflow tract. (LA, left atrium; LV, left ventricle; PA, pulmonary artery; RV, right ventricle.)

VI

Prosthetic Valvular Disease

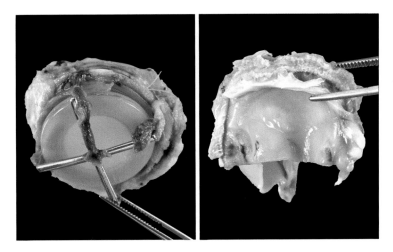

(Left) Starr-Edwards disc valve. A thrombus is visible on the stent.
(Right) Ionescu-Shiley pericardial xenograft. There is degeneration of
the valvular tissue adjacent to the stent, and a fissure has formed.

In serious valvular disease when medical therapy becomes difficult, the valve may be surgically repaired or replaced. In the former procedure, valve adhesions are manually stripped and opened. Since rheumatic valvular disease frequently involves adhesions of the commissures, this procedure is termed a *commissurotomy*. Recently, remarkable progress has also been made in valve replacement techniques.

There are three types of valves used in valve replacement: mechanical valves homograft (allograft) tissue valves, and heterograft (xenograft) tissue valves. In this chapter, these are classified and discussed as mechanical and tissue valves.

Tissue valves use valves and tissue from animals of the same or different species. Porcine aortic valves and bovine heart valves have been used frequently in recent years. A variety of mechanical valves are available. These include the Hufnagel ball valve, disc valves, the tilting disc valve (with fan-like movement designed to achieve maximal axial flow), and the St. Jude Medical valve (a new bi-leaflet valve). These valves are improving each year, with increasingly better surgical outcomes.

Tissue Valve Dysfunction

Tissue valves have been widely adopted for clinical applications because they tend to produce less thrombosis and provide better axial (central) flow than mechanical valves, and because after they are implanted they produce no noise associated with the heartbeat. The most important problems with tissue valves are poor durability and vulnerability to infection. There is no consensus on the number of years that tissue valves can be expected to last, but results in younger patients are said to be particularly unfavorable. The dysfunction most commonly seen in tissue valves is degenerative thickening of the valvular leaflets, leading to eventual rupture. Although attempts are being made to improve valve processing and manufacture, there is still considerable room for improvement.

Tissue valves are also prone to marked tissue degeneration of the valve itself. Fibrotic degeneration can lead to serious complications such as edema, deposition of degeneration products, and calcification. Not infrequently, further surgery is required to replace the original tissue valve. Left ventriculography can show mitral regurgitation; in the presence of perforations, such regurgitation often develops adjacent to the stent. In ventriculography, it is important to distinguish whether regurgitation is due to tissue valve dysfunction or to regurgitation in the valve periphery.

Findings from echocardiography include thickening of the valve, restricted opening due to sclerosis, valve fissuring, and fissure-induced prolapse of the valve. Dehiscence of the prosthetic valve from the peripheral tissue is also sometimes seen.

Using Doppler techniques, stenosis can be evaluated by measuring the maximum flow across the opening of the prosthetic valve. Valve dysfunction can be determined by detecting regurgitation. The point of origin of the regurgitation indicates whether this regurgitation is from within the prosthetic valve or from the valve periphery.

Although they are both tissue valves, porcine aortic valves develop dysfunction slowly, while among bovine heart valves there are instances in which the valve leaflets rupture suddenly; timing of further surgery must be carefully considered.

Pathologic and morphologic findings show (1) on gross examination, destruction of the valve itself at the periphery of the stent, accompanied by degenerative thickening (with xanthomas frequently present), and (2) histological degeneration of the collagen fibers that make up the valvular tissue, involving edema, deposition of degeneration products, and calcification.

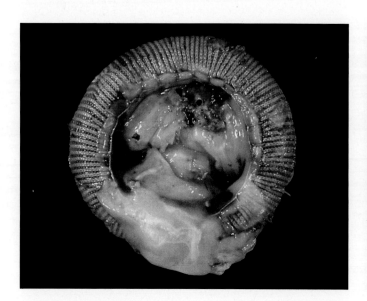

FIG. 236 Hancock valve dysfunction. The patient was a 30-year-old woman. There is prominent calcification of the valve leaflets.

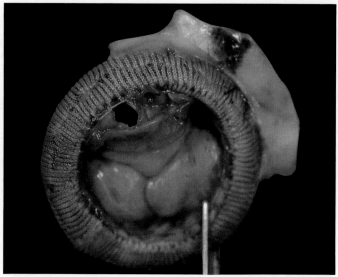

FIG. 237 Hancock valve dysfunction. The patient was a 43-year-old woman. There is dysfunction of this prosthetic valve with a notable perforation.

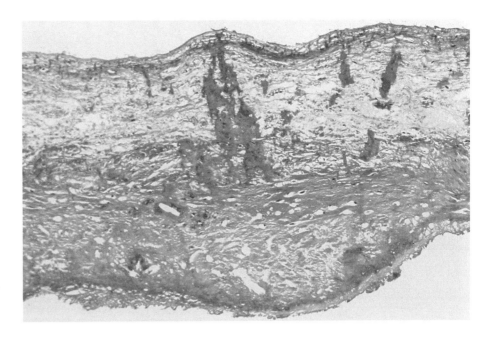

FIG. 238 Tissue section of a leaflet from a resected Hancock valve. The patient was a 48-year-old woman. At age 29, she developed left hemiparesis as a consequence of a cerebral embolism and at age 30, underwent a closed mitral valvular commissurotomy. At age 44, the mitral valve was replaced. One month previously, the patient developed dyspnea and heart failure. Echocardiography showed perforation of the Hancock valve, and a valve replacement procedure was performed. Marked degeneration of the collagen fibers of the valve leaflet and thinning and elongation of the leaflet are shown. Scattered calcified deposits are visible, and there is prominent monocytic infiltration on the surface of the leaflet. (HE stain, × 175.)

FIG. 239 Left ventriculography (30-degree right anterior oblique view). A perforation has developed in the superior part of the Ionescu-Shiley valve, with a wide regurgitant jet (black arrow) emitted against the anterior wall of the left atrium. (LA, left atrium; LV, left ventricle; rj, regurgitant jet.)

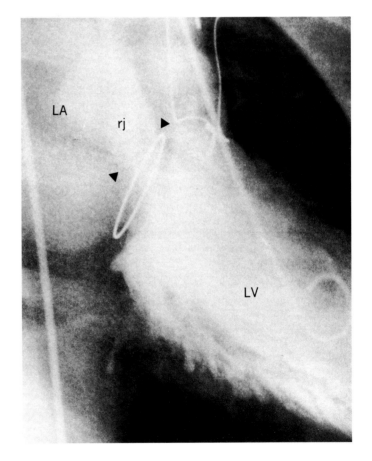

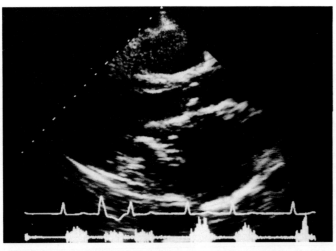

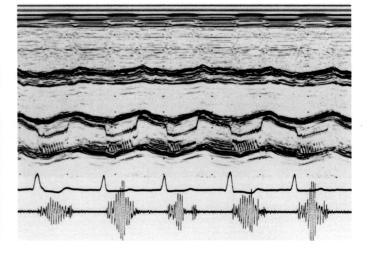

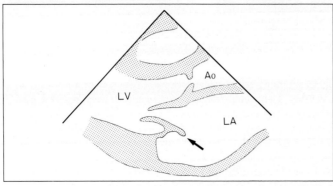

FIG. 240 Echocardiography. Hancock valve dysfunction. (Left) Cross-sectional echocardiography on the long axis shows a portion of the valve prolapsing into the left atrium (arrow). (Right) M-mode echocardiography shows fluttering of the damaged valve during systole. (Ao, aorta; LA, left atrium; LV, left ventricle.)

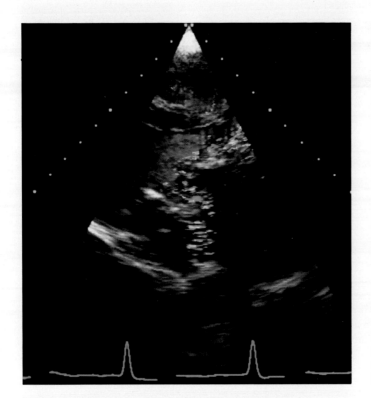

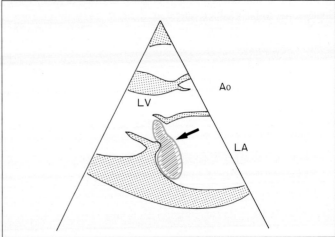

FIG. 241 Doppler imaging. A cross-section of the long axis of the left ventricle during systole. The stent of the prosthetic valve is visible at the mitral valve position. A regurgitant jet is evidenced from the medial aspect of the valvular ring to the left atrium. This mitral regurgitation was attributed to prosthetic valve dysfunction. (Ao, aorta; LA, left atrium; LV, left ventricle.)

Mechanical (Nontissue) Valve Dysfunction

Mechanical valve dysfunction is often caused by thrombus formation. Angiography makes it possible to identify the insufficiency as valvular regurgitation, which must be distinguished from regurgitation at the valve periphery. Restricted opening of ball valves and disc valves can be evaluated by fluoroscopy and/or cineangiography.

Echocardiography can reveal decreased mobility of the valve, abnormal echoes at the valve periphery (suggesting the possibility of thrombus), or the appearance of abnormal motion of the valve seat.

The onset of dysfunction in mechanical valves is rapid in comparison to tissue valves. Before the appearance of hemodynamically significant dysfunction, abnormalities of disc movement can be detected by echocardiography, phonocardiography, or fluoroscopy. Any changes in these findings require extremely close attention during long-term follow-up observation.

Pathologic and morphologic findings may include (1) adherent thrombi, (2) pannus formation, and (3) damage to the valve or its supporting structures.

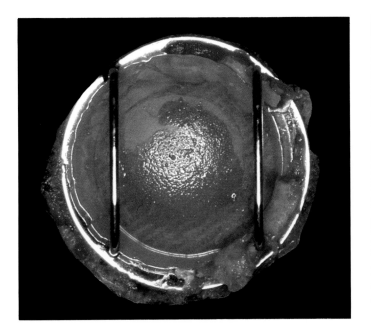

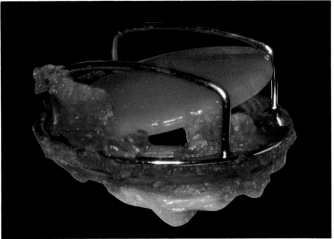

FIG. 243 Lateral view of the Kay-Shiley valve from the patient discussed in Fig. 242. Thrombotic vegetations extend from the valve ring to the supporting structures.

FIG. 242 View from the ventricular side of a Kay-Shiley valve implanted in the mitral valve position. The patient was a 46-year-old woman. At age 20, she was diagnosed with valvular disease and at age 25, underwent mitral valve replacement. One month previously, the patient experienced the onset of exertional dyspnea and underwent a second valve replacement. Thrombotic vegetations are attached to the valvular ring, and the disc margins are worn and irregular.

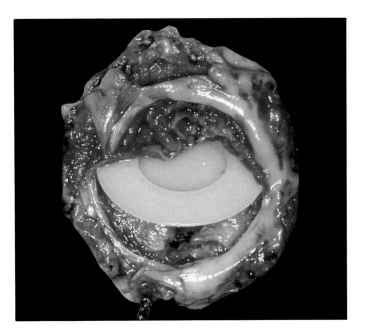

FIG. 244 View from the ventricular side of a Bjork-Shiley valve implanted in the aortic valve position. The patient was a 35-year-old woman. At age 25, she underwent replacement of the aortic valve because of rheumatic aortic stenosis. Approximately 1 month previously, the patient developed sudden dyspnea. The click sound of the prosthetic valve was sometimes inaudible, but there were no other remarkable changes. Twenty-three days previously, in the eighth month of pregnancy, valvular dysfunction was suspected, and the patient was admitted to the hospital for in-patient observation. One day previously, the click from the prosthetic valve weakened and aortic regurgitation increased. At this point, a second valve replacement was performed. The valve is covered by thrombus, and valve opening and closing is restricted.

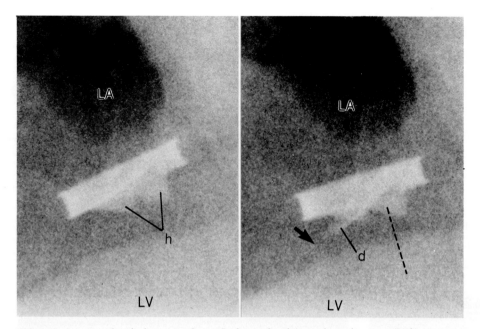

FIG. 245 Angiographic findings. An Omni-Carbon valve, hepatoclavicular view. (Left) During systole, the disc moves into the stent and cannot be seen. (Right) During diastole, the disc, which should open to a perpendicular position (dashed line), only moves to the tip of the black arrow, producing mitral valve stenosis. (d, disc; h, hinge; LA, left atrium; LV, left ventricle.)

Prosthetic Valve Endocarditis

Vegetations that are present on the heart valve because of prosthetic valve endocarditis are sometimes visible as relatively large filling defects in diagnostic imaging.

Echocardiography can show abnormal motion of the valve seat (particularly in mechanical valves), and valve thickening and vegetations in tissue valves.

In prosthetic valve endocarditis, medical therapy is more difficult than for infections in natural valves, enlargement of vegetations occurs earlier, and the incidence of embolic complications is high. In treatment, indications for surgical intervention should always be considered.

For a discussion of pathologic and morphologic findings, see Chapter 3, the section, Infectious Endocarditis.

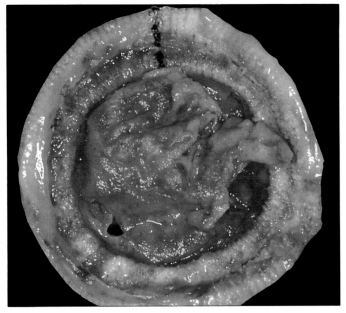

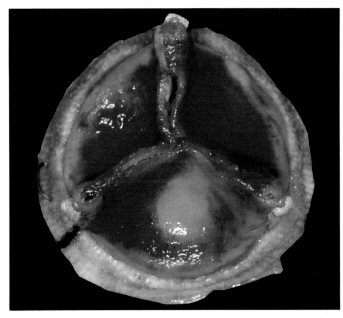

FIG. 246 View from the atrial side of an Ionescu-Shiley valve implanted in the mitral valve position. The patient was a 67-year-old man. Three years previously, he developed asthma-like symptoms and 2 years previously, began to experience dyspnea even when walking on level ground. The patient underwent mitral valve replacement 33 days previously, but a persistent postoperative fever developed. *Streptococcus faecalis* was isolated in blood cultures, and on that same day, a second valve replacement was performed. Most of the valvular orifice is covered with thrombotic vegetations. A valve leaflet perforation is visible near the ring.

FIG. 247 View from the ventricular side of the Ionescu-Shiley valve of the case discussed in Fig. 246. Thin thrombi are diffusely adherent to the valve leaflets.

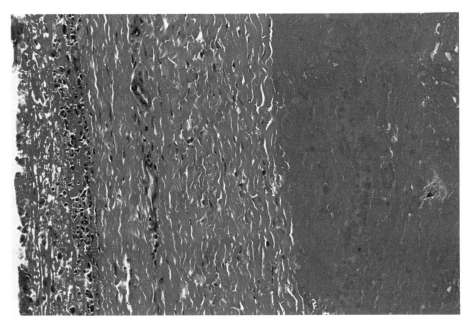

FIG. 248 Tissue section of a leaflet of the Ionescu-Shiley valve of the case discussed in Fig. 246. A thrombus is attached to the atrial surface, and neutrophilic and large monocytic infiltrations are visible. There is an additional thrombus on the ventricular surface, and numerous bacteria are visible near the valve leaflet. There is virtually no intrinsic degeneration of the valve leaflet. (HE stain, × 195.)

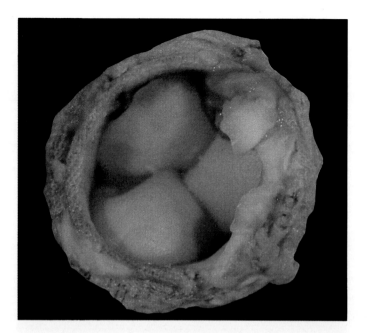

FIG. 249 View from the aortic side of an Ionescu-Shiley valve implanted in the aortic valve position. The patient was a 73-year-old man. At age 39, he developed symptoms of exertional dyspnea and at age 46, underwent a closed commissurotomy of the mitral valve. Sick sinus syndrome developed at age 66, followed at age 71 by the start of multiple attacks of Adams-Stokes syndrome. Six months previously, the aortic and mitral valves were replaced. Subsequently, the patient experienced repeated episodes of prosthetic valve endocarditis, necessitating a second replacement of the aortic valve. Spherical thrombotic vegetations are visible around the sutured regions of two valve leaflets.

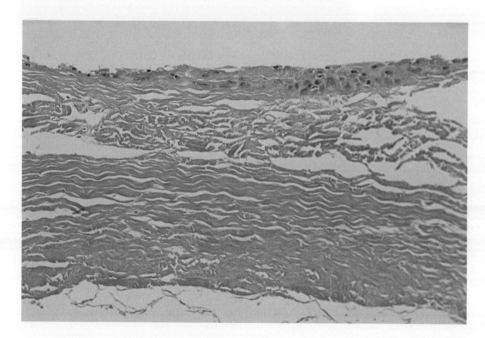

FIG. 250 Tissue section of a leaflet of the Ionescu-Shiley valve of the case discussed in Fig. 249. Infiltration by large monocytes is visible in the superficial layer of the valve. There is no apparent degeneration of the collagen fibers. (HE stain, × 50.)

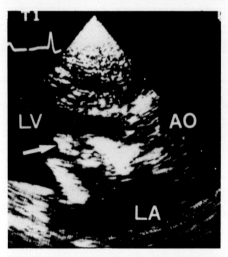

FIG. 251 Cross-sectional echocardiography on the long axis showing the presence of vegetations (acute phase). Vegetations are seen between the stents (arrow). (Ao, aorta; LA, left atrium; LV, left ventricle.)

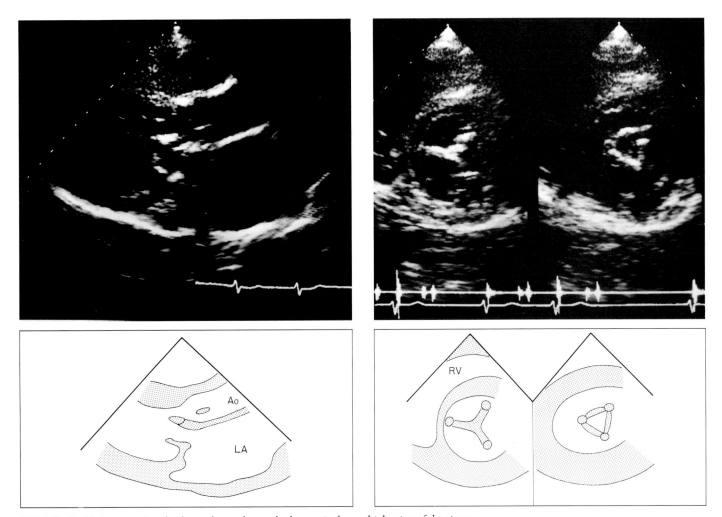

FIG. 252 (Left) Cross-sectional echocardiography on the long axis shows thickening of the tissue valve. (Right) Cross-sectional echocardiography on the short axis (left side shows valve closing, right side shows valve opening) reveals thickening of the three leaflets. (Ao, aorta; LA, left atrium; RV, right ventricle.)

Suggested Readings

Radiographic Inspection

1. Mezaros WT: Cardiac Roentgenology. Charles C Thomas, Springfield, IL, 1969

2. Jefferson K, Ree S: Clinical Radiology. Butterworths, London, 1973

3. McAlpine WA: Heart and Coronary Arteries. Springer, New York, 1975

4. Yang SS, Bentivoglio LG, Maranhao V, Goldberg H: From Cardiac Catheterization Data to Hemodynamic Parameters. 2nd. Ed. FA Davis, Philadelphia, 1978

5. Grossman W: Cardiac Catheterization and Angiography. 2nd. Ed. Lea & Febiger, Philadelphia, 1980

6. Kimata S, Momma K, Inoue Y: [Angiocardiography.] Igaku-shoin, Tokyo, 1981

7. Tasaka A (ed): [Encyclopedia of Clinical Radiology. Vol. 11.] Nakayama-Shoten, Tokyo, 1983

8. Tasaka A (ed): [Encyclopedia of Clinical Radiology. Vol. 12.] Nakayama-Shoten, Tokyo, 1985

9. Kozuka T, Nosaki T: [Cardiac Roentgenology.] Nanzando, Tokyo, 1985

10. Spindola-Franco H, Fish BG: Radiology of the Heart. Springer, New York, 1985

Ultrasound Inspection

11. Yoshikawa J: Cho-onpa Shinzo Danso-zu no Rinsho [Clinical Medicine: Two-Dimensional Ultrasonic Wave of Heart]. Kanehara, Tokyo, 1979

12. Machii K (ed): [Two-Dimensional Echocardiography.] Chugai Igaku, Tokyo, 1981

13. Miyatake K, Okamoto M, Kinoshita N et al: Pulmonary regurgitation studied with the ultrasonic pulsed Doppler technique. Circulation 65:969, 1982

14. Miyatake K, Okamoto M, Kinoshita N et al: Evaluation of tricuspid regurgitation by pulsed Doppler and two-dimensional echocardiography. Circulation 66:777–783, 1982

15. Nagata S, Nimura Y, Beppu S et al: Mechanism of systolic anterior motion of mitral valve and site of intraventricular pressure gradient in hypertrophic cardiomyopathy. Br Heart J 49:234, 1983

16. Nagata S, Nimura Y, Sakakibara H: Mitral valve lesion associated with secundum atrial septal defect. Analysis by real-time two-dimensional echocardiography. Br Heart J 49:51, 1983

17. Machi K (ed): Rinsho Danso-shin Echo Zu Handoku Koza [Textbook of Clinical Medicine: Two-dimensional Echocardiography, Vol 1). Kanehra, Tokyo, 1982

18. Omoto R: [Color Atlas of Real-Time Two-Dimensional Doppler Echocardiography.] Shindan-To-Chiryo, Tokyo, 1983

19. Miyatake K, Okamoto M, Kinoshita N et al: Clinical applications of new type of real-time two-dimensional flow imaging system. Am J Cardiol 54:857–868, 1984

20. Nagata S, Park Y-D, Nagae K et al: Echocardiographic feature of bioprosthetic valve endocarditis. Br Heart J 51:263, 1984

21. Hatle L, Angelsen B: Valve regurgitation. pp. 153–177. In: Doppler Ultrasound in Cardiology. Lea & Febiger, Philadelphia, 1985

22. Nanda NC: Doppler Echocardiography. Igaku-shoin, New York, 1985

23. Wagai T, Matsuo H (eds): Cho-onpa Igaku [Ultrasonic Medicine]. Nagai Shoten, Tokyo, 1985

24. Feigenbaum H: Echocardiography, 4th Ed. Lea & Febiger, Philadelphia, 1986

25. Kitabatake A, Inoue M (eds): [Textbook of Doppler Echocardiography.] Maruzen, Tokyo, 1986

26. Miyatake K, Izumi S, Okamoto M et al: Semiquantitative grading of severity of mitral regurgitation by real-time two-dimensional Doppler flow imaging technique. J Am Coll Cardiol 7:82–88, 1986

27. Miyatake K, Yamamoto K, Park Y-D et al: Diagnosis of mitral valve perforation by real-time two-dimensional Doppler flow imaging technique. J Am Coll Cardiol 8:1235–1239, 1986

28. Helmcke F, Nanda NC, Hsiung MC et al: Color Doppler assessment of mitral regurgitation with orthogonal planes. Circulation 75:175–183, 1987

29. Takahiro Kozuka (Ed): Clinical Diagnosis of the Heart by Imaging. Maruzen, Tokyo (1988) in Japanese

Pathology/Morphology

30. Gould SE: Pathology of the Heart and Blood Vessels. 3rd Ed. Charles C Thomas, Springfield, IL, 1968

31. Murao S (ed): [Valvular Heart Disease.] Nankodo, Tokyo, 1976

32. Pomerance A, Davies MJ: The Pathology of the Heart. Blackwell Scientific Publications, Oxford, 1975

33. Netter FH: Heart. The Ciba Collection of Medical Illustrations. Vol. V. CIBA, New York, 1978

34. Roberts WC: Congenital Heart Disease in Adults, FA Davis, Philadelphia, 1979

35. Davies MJ: Pathology of Cardiac Valves. Butterworths, London, 1980

36. Olsen EGJ: The Pathology of the Heart. 2nd Ed. Macmillan, London, 1980

37. Becker AE, Anderson RH: Cardiac Pathology. Gower Medical, New York, 1982

38. Sugiura M, Ohkawa S: [Atlas of Heart Disease in Old Age.] Nanzando, Tokyo, 1982

39. Silver MD: Cardiovascular Pathology. Churchill Livingstone, New York, 1983

40. Davies MJ: Cardiovascular Pathology. Harvey Miller, Oxford University Press, London, 1986

41. Olsen EGJ: Cardiovascular Pathology. MTP Press, Lancaster, 1987

42. Rose AG: Pathology of Heart Valve Replacement. MTP Press, 1987

43. Willerson JT, Cohn JN (eds): Cardiovascular Medicine. Churchill Livingstone, New York, 1995

Surgery

44. Kalmanson D: The Mitral Valve—A Pluridisciplinary Approach. Edward Arnold, London, 1976

45. Doty DB: Cardiac Surgery. Year Book Medical, Chicago, 1985

46. Abe H (ed): [Textbook of Cardiovascular Disease. Vol. 7. Surgical Treatment for Cardiovascular Diseases.] Maruzen, Tokyo, 1986

47. Starek PJK: Heart Valve Replacement and Reconstruction. Year Book Medical, Chicago, 1987

48. Willerson JT, Cohn JN, Manabe H, Yutani C (eds): Atlas of Ischemic Heart Disease. Churchill Livingstone, New York, 1996